Menopause
the Natural Way

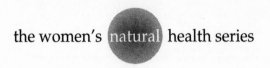

the women's natural health series

Menopause
the Natural Way

Deborah Gordon, M.D., Series Editor

MOLLY SIPLE, M.S., R.D.,
AND
DEBORAH GORDON, M.D.

A Lynn Sonberg Book

JOHN WILEY & SONS, INC.
New York • Chichester • Weinheim • Brisbane • Singapore • Toronto

ISBN: 0-471-37957-3

Printed in the United States of America

10 9 8 7 6 5 4 3 2 1

Important Note

This book is for informational purposes only. It is not intended to take the place of medical advice from a trained medical professional. Readers are advised to consult a physician or other qualified health professional regarding treatment of all of their health problems or before acting on any of the information or advice in this book.

This book is intended to provide selected information about menopause. Research about menopause is ongoing and subject to conflicting interpretations. As a result, there is no guarantee that what we know about this subject won't change with time.

Contents

INTRODUCTION
1

CHAPTER ONE
Welcome to Menopause, 5

CHAPTER TWO
Signs of Menopause, 17

CHAPTER THREE
Creating a Healthy and Empowering Passage
through Menopause: Getting Started on the
Six-Step Healthy Menopause Program, 35

CHAPTER FOUR
Step 1: Nutrients and Menopause—
Vitamins, Minerals, and Special Nutrients, 47

CHAPTER FIVE
Step 2: Diet and Menopause—The Way to Eat, 83

CHAPTER SIX
Step 3: Herbs and Menopause, 101

CHAPTER SEVEN

Step 4: Exercise and Menopause, 127

CHAPTER EIGHT

Step 5: Stress Management and Menopause, 145

CHAPTER NINE

Step 6: Hormone Replacement Therapy, 155

CHAPTER TEN

Staying Healthy as You Age, 179

GLOSSARY
205

SOURCES
209

RESOURCES
213

INDEX
231

Menopause
the Natural Way

...dictions. Men have even joined the conversation and begun to learn more about the women in their lives.

Many women are challenged or confront...

Introduction

By Deborah Gordon, M.D.

Whether menopause is years away or you are experiencing symptoms today, you should learn all you can about this natural life process. The more you know, the better you can take care of yourself. And the healthier you are, the easier your menopause is likely to be.

Over the centuries, women have privately conferred and shared information about remedies to ease symptoms of menopause. However, until recently these conversations took place behind closed doors. Menopause was a hush-hush subject. But with the help of the media, women broke the silence. Menopause has become the subject of the day and has been featured on television, in magazines, on Web sites, and in menopause newsletters. Men have even joined the conversation and have begun to learn more about the women in their lives.

Many women are challenged by menopause. Even if a woman does not have menopausal symptoms, the way she defines herself changes. I've had patients who are practically symptom-free, perhaps needing to be treated only for vaginal dryness and welcoming this new phase of life. They use menopause as an opportunity to reassess priorities and reevaluate their life.

1

For other patients, menopause is a wake-up call that prods them to take better care of their health. Just as many women are led to finally explore their artistic talents or go deeper into their spirituality at this time in life, menopause also stimulates women to take a closer look at their physical well-being. I believe that the greatest gift I can give these women is a properly selected homeopathic remedy to bring their health into balance and to allow their bodies to heal at the core. In addition, once I see that homeopathy is having a positive effect, I also advise them on diet, nutrition supplements, exercise, and stress management to help them maintain their health in the midst of life changes. Even when these women are no longer having obvious problems such as hot flashes, fatigue, and sleep disorder, and homeopathy is producing changes at a very fundamental level, living a healthy lifestyle remains vitally important.

I also have patients who, although they are taking a well-chosen homeopathic remedy and receiving the best advice about lifestyle, still require hormone replacement, either because they suffer from intolerable menopausal symptoms or are at high risk for osteoporosis. For these women, I make sure they understand their different hormone options. We then experiment with various regimens to find the best one for them. I also work with older woman, many years post-menopause, who are not taking hormones or are following a protocol I would not recommend. We talk and develop a program together. I invite all women to return with their problems, successes, and questions. Communication can be a powerful healing tool!

That is the reason this book was written—to communicate what's known about the treatments and medical recommendations for preventing and treating the symptoms of menopause. If you feel like a beginner, don't worry. You are not alone. Most women know very little about the change. Many who assume they are well informed often find out that what they have learned about menopause is not true, or at least not true for everyone. Women are not sure when menopause begins or what it feels like. They mistake signs of perimenopause for premenstrual syndrome (PMS). And some women are unclear about what menopause means in terms of their own life cycle. Is the change a brief transition, or is it the first stage of old age?

This book answers these questions and more. It also presents the Six-Step Healthy Menopause Program, which gives you these options:

1. Using nutrients to bolster health
2. Following a diet that supports female health
3. Taking herbs to allay symptoms
4. Exercising to ease symptoms and strengthen the body
5. Managing stress, which can exacerbate menopausal problems
6. Supplementing with hormones

Taking care of yourself through diet, exercise, and other natural means can be highly effective if you conscientiously stick to a plan. It requires discipline, but it's much better to support your health by following simple guidelines rather than dramatic intervention. For instance, heavy menstrual bleeding, which can occur during perimenopause, is sometimes treated with strong medications, repeated D&Cs (dilation and curettage), and even hysterectomy, although lifestyle modification can offer a solution that works for many women.

As you read through the following chapters and try out some of the recommendations, you may find that one or another of these approaches is all you need to make your symptoms manageable. Or you may need a combination of therapies to feel better. Of course, whatever treatments you decide to try, it's always a good idea to consult with a health professional. Search out someone with whom you feel comfortable and who can help guide you to make informed decisions about the particular type of treatment you require. There is no one way to handle menopause. You are unique and the way you manage your health must be individualized too.

CHAPTER ONE

Welcome to Menopause

In this chapter, we give you an introduction to menopause. We discuss how menopause has been viewed and defined by the medical establishment, as well as the effect of culture and society on the menopause experience. A brief biology lesson will give you the foundation for the options explained in subsequent chapters to manage the symptoms of menopause.

Types of Menopause

Menopause is a normal and universal event. It begins when you have not had a menstrual period for at least 1 full year. If you are female and live long enough, you will inevitably experience this change in hormone production. Clinicians differentiate between types of menopause. The expected cessation of menstruation at midlife is considered *natural menopause*. When periods stop because a woman has undergone an operation in which her ovaries are removed, this condition is referred to as *artificial* or *surgical menopause*. And *premature menopause* describes menopause that occurs before age 40, and from unknown causes. About 8% of women have a premature menopause.

Facts and Figures

Much data have been collected about when menopause is likely to occur, the number of women currently passing through menopause, and so forth. Here are some of the details:

- As the populous baby-boom generation ages, 3500 American women enter the menopausal years—ages 45 to 54—every day.

- Between 1990 and 2010, almost 40 million American women will pass through menopause.

- The average age of natural menopause is 51 to 52.

- By age 55, 95% of American women cease menstruating.

- As many as 25% of women report no discomfort during menopause. Only about 10 to 20% experience discomforts severe enough that they seek medical attention.

- Because women are healthier than they were in the past, they can expect to live one-third of their adult lives postmenopause.

- Although depression has been considered a sign of menopause, no clear causal relationship has been proven.

- Most women report that their sexual relations remain the same or even improve after menopause.

The Normal Menstrual Cycle

Women are lunar creatures. Our hormones ebb and flow according to a monthly rhythm. This rhythm directs the menstrual cycle that occurs approximately every 28 days.

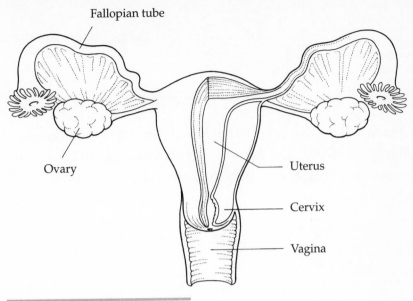

Female Reproductive Organs

The ovaries produce eggs. Every woman has a predetermined number from birth—about 100,000 to 400,000. They are in an inactive form, called a follicle. Hormones produced by the pituitary gland in the brain, follicle-stimulating hormone (FSH) and luteinizing hormone (LH), stimulate the follicles to ripen to produce a fully developed egg. The maturing follicle also begins to produce the two sex hormones, estrogen and progesterone. These hormones prepare the egg to be fertilized but also ready the uterus. Estrogen, which dominates for the first half of the menstrual cycle and declines after ovulation, causes the uterine lining to thicken. Progesterone, which dominates during the second half of the cycle, triggers changes in the uterus to provide a safe haven for a fertilized egg to mature into a fetus.

Only one egg is expelled from the ovaries and has the chance to come in contact with a sperm. If this occurs, the two unite and conception occurs. However, if the egg and the sperm miss each other, the uterus sheds its lining. The substances

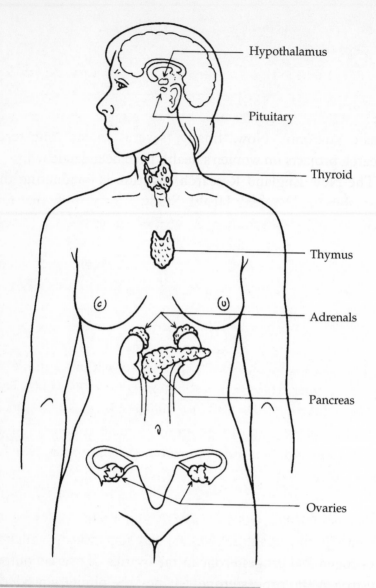

Glands and Organs Influencing Menopause

sloughed off, cells and blood that were meant to nourish the fetus, are known as menstrual flow.

This sequence of events occurs over a month's time, and if conception does not take place, the cycle begins again.

RESEARCH INTO FEMALE HEALTH: PLAYING CATCH-UP

The great majority of research done on human health has focused on males, not females. Some anatomy books at the turn of the 20th century did not even include illustrations of female anatomy. Now, finally, several major long-term research projects on women's health have been launched.

The New England Research Institute is conducting the Massachusetts Women's Health Study, a large study that follows the health of middle-aged women over a 7-year period, focusing on perimenopause and related symptoms. The National Institute of Aging has begun a study that will follow women as they go through menopause. And the National Institutes of Health has launched a massive national research effort to learn more about the causes of disease and death in middle-aged and older women, including heart disease, cancer, osteoporosis, and depression.

Dancing Hormones

Follicle-stimulating hormone (FSH) and luteinizing hormone (LH) are produced in the pituitary and help direct production of estrogen and progesterone in the ovaries. If ovarian output of estrogen and progesterone declines, the pituitary produces more FSH and LH to stimulate and increase production of these two important sex hormones. They are linked in a negative feedback system. If estrogen and progesterone output is excessive, less FSH and LH are produced. This coordinated system is designed to support the development of the egg, fertilization, and implantation of the egg into the wall of the uterus, and to sustain the early stages of pregnancy.

Hormones are powerful compounds because they are chemical messengers. Glands secrete these messenger compounds, which then enter the bloodstream. Hormones are keyed to certain target tissues. When circulating hormones arrive at their destination, they bind to receptor sites, like a key fitting into a lock. This sends a message to the target tissue, which may be another gland. The hormone will trigger the gland to release its own hormone or may directly trigger some chemical reaction. Some hormones cause changes within target tissues in just a few seconds, whereas the effects of others may be felt for days, weeks, or even years. The net effect is that hormones balance and pace various processes within the body.

Sex hormones are called steroid hormones. The major sex hormones are estrogen, progesterone, and testosterone, which are all made by both men and women but in different proportions. In women, estrogen and progesterone are essential for normal reproduction and the menstrual cycle.

Sex hormones are all derived from cholesterol. If you go on a low-fat diet, you may end up with such a low cholesterol level that your production of estrogen and progesterone declines. This is exactly what happens to teenage girls who diet and exercise to become very slim. By losing body fat, they may stop having periods. Conversely, women who are overweight tend to produce extra hormones, which is possibly why carrying extra pounds can be a risk factor for breast cancer.

Hormone Changes in Perimenopause

Here's how it all begins. Around age 40, the ovaries become less and less efficient and produce decreasing amounts of estradiol, the primary form of estrogen a woman's body produces, and progesterone, triggering a disruption in the cycle. This causes an increase in the production of FSH and LH in an effort to stimulate the ovaries to produce greater amounts of hormones.

As the ovaries and pituitary gland attempt to communicate and adjust, the ovaries may briefly and erratically produce excessive amounts of estrogen or progesterone. Then production will drop again. These highs and lows of hormone levels can lead to PMS-like symptoms, which are typical of perimenopause, the transitional phase that precedes menopause. Perimenopause typically begins 4 to 5 years before the menstrual cycle stops, on average at age 47½. Estrogen may dominate, then progesterone, each triggering certain symptoms. In perimenopause, the ovaries may not produce an egg during certain months and a woman will have an *anovulatory* cycle. If there is no ovulation, no progesterone is produced. This can result in an irregular and heavy menstrual cycle, typical of perimenopause. However, about 10% of women do not really have a perimenopausal phase and instead abruptly cease menstruation.

Estrogen Production Before and After Menopause

Before menopause the ovaries are the primary site of sex hormone production, including estrogen, progesterone, and testosterone. Most of the estrogen produced by the ovaries is in the form known specifically as 17ß-estradiol. This type of estrogen makes up 95% of the estrogen circulating in the blood.

With menopause, synthesis of estrogen by the ovaries declines. Estrogen output drops to 40% of premenopausal rates in women 50 to 60 years old and to 20% in most women older than 65. Although the amount is reduced, postmenopausal women do continue to produce some estrogen— a fact that is not appreciated or well understood. One study of

100 postmenopausal women found that the ovaries secrete some estrogens, although relatively small amounts, during the first 4 years postmenopause.

In addition, the adrenal glands function in postmenopause as a natural backup system for estrogen production. The adrenals produce an estrogen precursor, *androstenedione*, which is converted into another form of estrogen, *estrone*. Estrone is a less potent form of estrogen than estradiol. Estrone is mostly formed in the fatty tissue of the lower abdomen, but some is also produced in muscle tissue and bone marrow. In postmenopause the liver converts some estrone to a third configuration of estrogen, *estriol*.

The Social Side of Menopause

Ask any woman and she will tell you that menopause is a life event, full of meaning, a challenge psychologically and socially. For starters, negative attitudes toward menopause and menopausal women have persisted for hundreds of years and have been recorded in medical writing and found throughout literature. These indictments can make menopause feel like a burden, even if a woman isn't troubled by symptoms.

In the late 1700s, as treatments for menopause began to appear in the medical literature, the negative attitudes toward this stage of life showed up in the medical language.

In a treatise on female health in 1845, Colombat de L'Isere wrote:

> Compelled to yield to the power of time, women now cease to exist for the species, and hence forward live only for themselves. Their features are stamped with the impress of age, and their genital organs are sealed with the signet of sterility. . . . It is the dictate of prudence to avoid all such circumstances as might tend to awaken any erotic thoughts in the mind and reanimate a sentiment

that ought rather to become extinct . . . in fine, everything calculated to cause regret for charms that are lost, and enjoyments that are ended forever.

In recent times, too, medical literature has painted a grim picture of menopause. In 1963, in an article published in the *Journal of the American Geriatric Society*, entitled, "The Fate of the Nontreated Postmenopausal Woman. A Plea for the Maintenance of Adequate Estrogen from Puberty to the Grave," the authors wrote that, at menopause, "women acquired a vapid, cow-like feeling called a negative state in which the world appears as through a gray veil, and they live as docile, harmless creatures."

And an article in the same journal, in 1967, included the following: "Many women are leading an active and productive life when this tragedy strikes. They are still attractive and mentally alert. They deeply resent what to them is a catastrophic attack upon their ability to earn a living and enjoy life."

Even today, such terms as "ovarian failure" and "vaginal atrophy" are used to describe the change. It is no wonder that many women worry about menopause and fear it. Companies selling products for treatment of menopausal symptoms often make use of these dismal images to help sell their products. Here is a case in point.

Marilyn, a professional and single woman living in New York, found herself in a surgeon's office after being told she needed a full hysterectomy for fibroid removal; this surgery results in medically induced menopause. While waiting for her appointment in the clinic's reception area, she thumbed through the only reading material available—promotional literature from a drug company. The brochure informed her that once a woman is menopausal, her vaginal tissues soon become parched and withered, and intercourse is then difficult if not painful. The unstated subtext was only too clear to Marilyn— that from now on, if any man decided to go out with her, it would be an act of charity! She could kiss her love life good-bye, as well as any prospects of marriage. Marilyn recalls being ushered into the doctor's office and discussing the details of her coming surgery feeling as if she were being prepared for her exit from life!

Menopause Is Linked to Culture

The attitudes you have toward menopause have been, at least in part, shaped by your world. The culture in which you live, what your mother told you about menopause, what your friends say about it, the messages you hear through the media, all shape what menopause means to you.

Sociologists have studied this aspect of menopause, investigating the effect that society and culture have on a woman's experience of the change. In countries where women gain in status at midlife, such as in India, many women report having a relatively uneventful menopause and rarely suffer psychological symptoms. In these societies, older women are appreciated for the wisdom of their years and are considered an asset to society.

In Japan, too, menopause is colored by the culture in which it exists. In this society, driven by the work ethic, menopause problems are often viewed as a luxury disease of modernity, affecting women with too much time on their hands.

And in North America, where menopausal women sometimes experience a drop in status or simply become invisible, menopause is rarely welcomed. The culture celebrates and values youthfulness. Many women, themselves products of the culture, are very sensitive to this attitude. If at the same time children leave home, or husband and wife divorce, the menopausal years become all the more difficult. In these circumstances, the physical and emotional problems a woman has that can be attributed to menopause become difficult to define. Life and the change are intertwined.

Getting On with Your Life

Fortunately, many women are working hard to retire the images of the incapacitated menopausal woman. Women in their 60s go back to school to begin a second career. Many women work energetically well past an expected retirement age. Grandmothers hike up mountains. Sex symbols like Sophia Loren tell their age and smile at us from magazine covers. What's to fear, they ask. Get on with the rest of your life.

With menopause, women reach a plateau. For decades prior to menopause, women live a cyclical life, with steadily rising, then falling hormone levels. Now with menopause, their hormone levels become relatively steady, with the total output declining slowly over several years. Many women report finding new reserves of energy—what anthropologist Margaret Mead referred to as "postmenopausal zest."

The French have an expression that, roughly translated, means being comfortable in your own skin, which is a good way to go through menopause, in a spirit of self-acceptance. Some women resist menopause, although their body is sending all sorts of messages that a process of change has begun. It is better to face menopause head-on, like a sailboat cutting through the waves. You create less turbulence, you save energy, and you may reach the other side of menopause that much quicker.

Christiane Northrup, M.D., noted author and founder of the Women-to-Women health clinic in Yarmouth, Maine, points out, "The women now approaching menopause are part of the generation that were taught they couldn't trust any normal process of the body. They learned that menstrual flow must be controlled, and God forbid, someone should see a soiled sanitary napkin in the trash can! Even our mothers were systematically taught that breast feeding was not OK." But she offers another option: "Menopause can be a time of rebirth and redoing yourself from the inside out. By trusting the process, you can give yourself a smoother transition and emerge on the other side with everything intact and without delay."

In addition, accepting menopause can help you let go of your past and give you the opportunity of inventing a new and even grander you! So what are you waiting for? Take action and start by learning more about the signs and symptoms of menopause, the subject of the next chapter.

CHAPTER TWO

Signs of Menopause

When you hear the word *menopause*, do you cringe in anticipation of the symptoms? With all the publicity about menopause in the last few years, you probably are aware that a change in hormones can bring on such annoyances as hot flashes, mood swings, and occasional lapses of memory. However, problems like these are not inevitable, and when they do occur, they vary greatly in severity not only from woman to woman but from culture to culture.

Menopause in Other Cultures

The Japanese experience of menopause has been the subject of much study. A survey completed in 1983–84 interviewed over 1300 female factory workers and farm workers, as well as housewives. Among these women, only 9.7% reported having a hot flash in the 2 years immediately prior to menopause, and only 3.6% had night sweats. Of note is that there is no word for "hot flash" in the Japanese language. (The Chinese do not have a word for this symptom either.)

In contrast, some symptoms of menopause that are common in Japan rarely trouble North American women. At least these annoyances are not attributed to menopause. Typical Japanese complaints include shoulder and neck stiffness, dizziness, ringing in the ears, and unspecified aches and pains.

Menopause in Indonesian women also differs from the Western experience. An extensive study conducted in Indonesia found that nearly 80% of rural and uneducated women living in Central Java never experienced hot flashes. And according to other studies, women in many parts of the world, including India, Pakistan, Israel, Iraq, and Greece, describe menopause with far fewer hot flashes than the North American norm and a lower incidence of other symptoms as well.

There is even evidence that non-Western women are less affected by surgically induced menopause, which involves hysterectomy with removal of the ovaries, a procedure that usually produces acute symptoms. A study published in 1994, in the journal *Maturitas*, studied Chinese women in Hong Kong who had undergone this surgery. Less than 25% of these women reported having hot flashes compared with about 85% of North American women with surgically induced menopause.

Why Menopause Symptoms May Differ

Researchers have identified many factors that may determine a woman's individual experience of menopause. Whether or not a woman has become pregnant and how many children she has had may be a factor. Pregnancy and breast feeding suppress ovulation and estrogen production and may alter her estrogen profile at menopause. Such variations in the pattern of hormone production may influence which menopausal symptoms are likely to occur and their frequency.

Psychological factors may also color your experience of menopause. In some societies, women gain in status as they pass through menopause and enter a new phase of their life. A study of Sikh Indian women in Canada found that they looked forward to this time in life as being freeing and cleansing. At midlife, a Sikh woman begins to play a more prestigious role within her family and is regarded as an elder who has earned respect. Menopause is considered natural, requiring no special attention, and any discomforts that occur are more likely to be taken in stride. Few symptoms are reported, because they do not occur or because they are attributed to other causes, in this way supporting the belief that life is better.

Another theory, proposed by medical anthropologist Yewoubdar Beyene, Ph.D., is that the number of children a woman has had plays a role in menopausal symptoms. She suggests that some women have fewer symptoms because they married younger and gave birth to more children. Multiple pregnancies and breast feeding for a length of time change the pattern of hormone production over many years. Dr. Beyene has studied the menopausal experience in Greek and Mayan women. Dr. Beyene points out:

> There's a biocultural basis for symptoms American women are experiencing. American women typically marry late, have only one or two children, and either don't breast feed or only for a short period of time. Women elsewhere have a high reproduction rate and, cumulatively, a long period of lactation. Consequently, women in the West experience a relatively stable cycling of estrogen for most of their reproductive years. Then at menopause this stability is disrupted and the imbalance of hormones is felt more dramatically, perhaps triggering hot flashes and other symptoms.

And she continues:

> I don't like the current attitude that women are doomed by virtue of being women. What is really going on is that

western women have rapidly changed their lifestyles, while female biology has remained the same. I'm not saying we should all be having six to eight children, but if women realize that their experience of menopause is influenced by how they've chosen to live, symptoms of menopause may be easier to accept.

The foods a woman eats influence how her body adjusts to the change. Women in less developed areas of the world eat a more traditional diet than in the West. Food is less refined and processed and retains more of its original nutrients. Diets include an abundance of plant foods that supply phytoestrogens, which help balance hormones. Chapters 4 and 5 cover the subject of diet and nutrition in detail.

Stress also plays a role in symptoms. Some studies show that women in other countries who live in urban settings and lead a more modern lifestyle are more troubled by menopause than their rural counterparts. As explained in Chapter 8, stress can bring on and intensify many menopause symptoms.

Such diversity of experience is encouraging news. Menopausal signs are not inevitable. You may well have an easier time passing through this natural transition if you have been taking care of your health in the years leading up to menopause.

A SYMPTOM OR A SIGN?

In common parlance, the physical and emotional manifestations of menopause are referred to as "symptoms." Unfortunately, the term *symptom* implies that menopause is a disease, which it is not. We may, alternatively, think of the fallout from menopause as "signs." When a young woman begins to develop breasts, we say that this is a sign that her body is physically maturing. Likewise, when a woman at midlife ceases menstruating, this menopausal experience is a sign that she is passing into another phase of life.

Overview of the Signs of Menopause

This section describes various signs of menopause—what they actually feel like, their prevalence, and their origins and causes. You may already be having some of these symptoms, but you won't necessarily have them all. As you read through the following pages, remember that these descriptions are meant to help you maneuver through menopause, but they are not predictions!

Being better informed about the signs of menopause can help you deal with these new experiences. Having a little knowledge can even help reduce stress, which in itself can bring on symptoms.

Hot Flashes

The first time you have a hot flash can be quite disconcerting. With your first one, you probably won't even realize it's a hot flash. You may be sitting in your usual restaurant sipping a glass of wine when suddenly you want to fling off your clothes. Or you may be driving a car when another driver crowds you out of your lane. You may become annoyed, and, surprisingly, very hot. It's winter, but you open all the car windows so that you can breathe. That's a hot flash! Although the experience may feel strange and you may think you are sick, hot flashes are not life-threatening!

Taking in substances that stimulate the system, such as alcohol and coffee, as well as reacting to everyday stresses such as traffic, can trigger a hot flash. A wave of heat passes over your face and down your neck, or the heat works its way upward, starting in your upper torso and moving to your neck and head. It may feel like you are hot all the way through, but if you were to take your temperature it would be normal. The deep tissues of your body are not overheating. During a hot flash, only the outer layers of you are cooking! Skin temperature can increase as much as 7°, and, if you looked in the mirror, you'd see that your complexion had become red and flushed.

Next your body tries to cool down by generating perspiration. As your skin becomes damp, the perspiration evaporates into the air, naturally cooling the skin. This mechanism is so effective that you are likely to feel chilled. A hot flash can give you good reason to shed your jacket and 5 minutes later put it on again. Just a few years ago, having a hot flash in public was not socially acceptable and was a great embarrassment to many women. Fortunately, these days women do not feel as compelled to hide these changes in body temperature. Some have even learned to ride them out as validating "power surges." Give this approach a try when you have your next hot flash. You have nothing to lose. Assume that your body is behaving as it should, out of some form of inner guidance. See if you can discover for yourself what your body is trying to accomplish as it heats up.

Some women report experiencing heart palpitations during menopause. While these may be a new and unfamiliar experience, they are not usually cause for alarm, especially if they occur at the same time you are having a hot flash. However, you should immediately report to your physician heart palpitations that seem to come from nowhere. This phenomenon can be a symptom of more serious medical problems.

HOT-FLASH TIMING

About 65 to 75% of menopausal women experience hot flashes. For about half of these women, hot flashes begin during perimenopause as the menstrual cycle becomes irregular. Most of the remaining women report hot flashes within a year of menopause, but a small number of women have their first flash more than 2 years after menopause. Women report that hot flashes are most annoying during the first 2 years postmenopause. Having just a few hot flashes a day is most typical. However, this can vary from dozens each day to just a few per year. Most hot flashes last from 3 to 5 minutes, but can be as short as a few seconds. In general, they become less frequent and less intense with time. Taking hormone replacement therapy can greatly reduce or eliminate hot flashes and a diet high in certain nutrients can also reduce their frequency.

HOT-FLASH CHEMISTRY

The physiological causes of hot flashes are not thoroughly understood. The hypothalamus within the brain is certainly involved, since one of its functions is to regulate body temperature. But the hypothalamus can also alter regional blood flow, perhaps playing a role in bringing blood to surface skin tissue, thereby causing the typical hot-flash flushing. In addition, the hypothalamus serves as a link or bridge between the endocrine (hormonal) system and the nervous system. Alterations in the function of the hypothalamus can affect metabolic rate, sleep patterns, and sex drive, perhaps contributing to such midlife changes as weight gain, fatigue, and lowered libido.

Estrogen also plays a role in the process that can bring on a flash. Estrogen has an effect on both the hypothalamus and on norepinephrine, a stress hormone. Norepinephrine affects temperature regulation and the relationship between the endocrine and nervous systems. Low estrogen levels may affect the metabolism of norepinephrine, but rapidly changing estrogen levels—peaks and dips typical of perimenopause—may also be a factor.

Another theory is that low levels of estrogen are not as important as the withdrawal from estrogen. Dr. Fredi Kronenberg, in a paper published in 1990 in the *Annals of the New York Academy of Science*, points out that girls have low estrogen levels before they have had their first menstrual cycle, but they do not experience hot flashes. Women during pregnancy, when estrogen levels are high, report having hot flashes occasionally. Dr. Kronenberg suggests that declining estrogen levels that trigger a withdrawal reaction may be a more significant factor in the occurrence of hot flashes.

Perspiration Can Bring Inspiration

Besides sweating, hot flashes can trigger anxiety, irritation, and even panic. If you think you are having a panic attack, wait until your hot flash subsides before diagnosing yourself! Some women consider these emotional flare-ups a bonus. What you're feeling may give you useful insights into what needs changing in your life. You can take advantage of these moments. You'll probably thank yourself for not immediately acting on your feelings, but you may discover thoughts and ideas that need to be expressed. Try using your hot-flash thinking to reshape your life.

Night Sweats

If you have a hot flash during the night, you will experience night sweats. Menopausal women are frequently troubled by fatigue due to night sweats, which can occur many times throughout the night and can deprive women of REM (rapid eye movement) sleep during which dreaming occurs. Loss of REM is associated with a greater likelihood of feeling depressed.

To reduce night sweats, wear a thin cotton nightgown and make up your bed with several layers of lightweight bed linens. Remove these or layer them as your body temperature rises and falls.

SWEET DREAMS

Night sweats can disturb sleep. To help you go to sleep again, eat a small portion of cereal. The starches break down into sugars that increase your supply of serotonin, a neurotransmitter that helps regulate sleep. Sugar works the same way.

You can also supplement with melatonin, a hormone that regulates the sleeping/waking cycle. However, you need to take melatonin under the supervision of your health care practitioner. Alternatively, you can increase your body stores of this natural hormone by eating more foods that supply melatonin. These include oats, rice, sweet corn, tomatoes, and bananas.

Fatigue

Feeling tired is one of the most common menopausal symptoms. Menopause involves biological changes in various systems within the body. These alterations place a demand on energy. In addition, hot flashes can be exhausting, especially if they are accompanied by profuse sweating. As the body loses fluids as well as the essential minerals in these fluids, including sodium, potassium, and magnesium, you may feel drained of energy, just as a runner does after finishing a race. And, as already mentioned, night sweats are particularly tiring and can disrupt normal function. Studies show that even the loss of one night's sleep can result in tiredness, irritability, inability to concentrate, and mood swings. These annoyances are considered signs of menopause, but they may be due simply to sleep deprivation.

With menopause, many women find themselves longing for an afternoon nap. Madeleine, a manager of a busy clothing store, noticed that her energy level had begun to decline about the time she turned 49. She had been having irregular periods for a while and had also begun to experience hot flashes. Working on her feet for most of the day was now particularly tiring. At first she tried to push through her tiredness. However, the quality of her work began to suffer. Being a good supervisor of others, she decided to use her management skills on herself. Every afternoon at 3:00, Madeleine gave herself a half-hour break during which she sat down in a comfortable chair for some quiet time. She experimented with listening to soothing music, and practiced some breathing and meditation exercises. On most days, by 3:30 she was back in action with enough energy to finish her work. Madeleine is now well through menopause and is no longer experiencing such drops in energy. However, she learned from her experience. Madeleine now makes a point of giving other women on her staff the same freedom to take breaks when they need to.

Menopausal fatigue in most cases will subside as a woman's body adjusts to lower levels of hormones. However, if fatigue is related to a nutrient-poor diet, fundamental changes in eating habits need to take place before energy can substantially be restored. A diet of refined and processed foods often lacks sufficient B complex vitamins, potassium, magnesium, iron, iodine, and chromium, all nutrients required to maintain energy levels. Hypothyroidism, a condition in which the rate at which food is converted into energy has slowed, can also result in persistent fatigue. (See Chapter 10 for more information on menopause and thyroid function.)

Mood Swings

When the menopausal woman is caricatured, she's usually portrayed as moody, with emotions ranging from depression to irritability and rage. It is no surprise that many women anticipate menopause as one long siege of PMS mood swings.

During perimenopause, mood swings are typical just as they are in premenstrual syndrome. High levels of estrogen, relative to progesterone, which can occur at this time, can trigger anxiety and irritability, while high levels of progesterone, relative to estrogen, can bring on tearfulness. These two sex hormones have a profound effect on the function of the central nervous system, and imbalances can lead to emotional highs and lows. Night sweats can also cause irritability as they disrupt refreshing sleep.

Anger

With the onset of menopause, some women begin to feel an anger, even rage, that is quite unfamiliar. This powerful emotion, which a woman may have repressed over the years for a variety of reasons such as keeping the peace at home, now suddenly surges forth. Spontaneously feeling rage can be quite a surprise! A small, everyday annoyance that could at one time be taken in stride may now trigger an outburst.

Before you try to sweep these feelings under the carpet, take a moment and notice what you are crying over. Try to figure out why you've raised your voice. You may be experiencing an exaggerated reaction to some upset, but your anger may be sending you a message. If what you're thinking feels true for you, try communicating your thoughts with those individuals closest to you. Sharing your thoughts has the potential of improving your relationships and increasing intimacy.

Jeannine, who describes herself as a typical housewife, used menopause as the catalyst for speaking out. One day, while clearing the dishes from the table after a meal, she was suddenly overtaken with a welling up of feeling. She was walking, silverware in hand, through the door of her kitchen when, instead of calmly taking the silverware to the sink, she found herself spontaneously flinging forks and knives across the room in the general direction of the kitchen counter! As Jeannine recalls, "I had no idea why I was suddenly doing this, but it felt great! It was so untypical of me, I burst out laughing." When she calmed down, she began to wonder what this outburst was about. Jeannine began to think about all the household chores she was so very tired of doing and other aspects of her life that she really wanted to change.

She decided to tell her family members what was brewing, but didn't know how to go about this. She wisely consulted a family counselor before really opening up, to keep from placing blame on everyone and making the situation worse. Jeannine remembers, "My dear husband and children listened with some surprise to my newly expressed needs and wishes, but also with appreciation." Now she brags, "I was able to let things out. And as I showed up more as myself, I actually gave my family a chance to become closer to me. Out of this experience, my husband and I reinvented our marriage, and we've never gotten along so well. I'd advise any woman—when you are feeling ready to burst, go for it!"

Depression

Normal menopause is not likely to trigger depression. Having a full hysterectomy, in which the ovaries are removed, is a risk factor, as is having a history of depression. However, population studies consistently show that women are most likely to suffer from depression in their 20s and 30s, not at midlife. Moreover, neither suicides nor psychiatric hospitalizations increase among women in their late 40s or early 50s.

Weight Gain

A woman's metabolism is likely to slow down as she approaches midlife. This is one reason women normally gain 5 to 6 additional pounds as they pass through the change. In addition, fluid retention during perimenopause may help tip the scales. The body's normal regulation of water balance can become disturbed. Extracellular fluid accumulates, resulting in edema and sudden weight gain.

Changes in hormone production also lead to changes in body size and shape. In a study published in 1992 in the *Amer-*

ican Journal of Clinical Nutrition, among 131 women, ages 19 to 63, postmenopausal women were found to have 20% more fat than premenopausal women.

This increase in fat serves a purpose. In effect, at menopause, fat is virtually a sex organ! As production of estrogen by the ovaries declines, the fatty tissue of a woman's belly becomes an important site for estrogen production.

A Change in Profile

At midlife, a woman's fat begins to redistribute itself, following a pattern more typical of men. This reflects changes in her hormone production, as female sex hormones decline and testosterone makes up a greater percentage of hormone output. Women lose lower body fat, particularly in the hips and thighs, but gain upper body fat. These changes can be a health concern, as upper body fat is associated with a greater risk of heart disease. Going on a diet may be appropriate, but menopause is not the time to attempt a radical diet. If you try to cut back on calories, make sure you still take in sufficient nutrients, which your body especially needs to help adapt to the changes taking place.

Memory Loss

Dorothy, a housewife and the mother of two teenage girls, found herself waking up in the middle of the night, unable to remember the names of her children! Such dismaying and even humorous lapses of memory can begin occurring in the years leading up to menopause. When you telephone someone, you may find that by the time the person answers, you've forgotten whom you've called. No, this isn't a sign that you've suddenly become senile. Your brain is simply in a period of adjustment to changes in the amounts of sex hormones you are producing.

Poor verbal memory may be due to general changes in the central nervous system associated with aging. However, researchers also believe that declining estrogen levels interfere with verbal memory. It appears that estrogen may affect certain brain enzymes, that alter the metabolism of acetylcholine, a primary neurotransmitter considered critical to memory function. At the same time, estrogen levels appear to have no effect on spatial memory.

Fortunately, these lapses tend to diminish as you move through menopause. Being postmenopausal does not mean that you will be troubled by poor short-term memory forever. However, exercising your brain is absolutely necessary. Go out of your way to use your memory in order to sharpen your recall. Dare yourself to go to the supermarket without a shopping list! Go to a party and practice remembering people's names.

Brain Fog

In addition to actual memory lapses, certain fuzzy-headedness can crop up with menopause. A vagueness can set in that can disrupt your functioning, particularly if you have a demanding job that requires crisp thinking. Low estrogen levels may bring this on, and again, this symptom tends to clear up as you emerge on the other side of menopause.

Women understandably try to clear up their brain fog. Caffeine is often the drug of choice, in coffee, teas, and colas. Better ways include increasing the amount of water you drink, exercising more, eating a more nutritious diet that includes B vitamins and essential fatty acids, and experimenting with supplemental hormones—approaches outlined in this book.

But there is another, more positive way to look at brain fog. Perhaps brain fog is, for some women, an indication that the way they think is changing. In our society, women are encouraged to think like men, in a linear fashion. But as they pass through menopause, perhaps they naturally shift away from this thinking style and move toward a more intuitive way of comprehending.

Sexuality and Menopause

While menopause marks the end of a woman's reproductive years, a woman's sexuality does not vanish along with her ability to reproduce. In fact, one-third of postmenopausal women report no change in their sex lives and another third say that their sexual experiences have actually improved. They no longer are bothered by messy periods, they enjoy more privacy once children have moved out of the house, and they have more leisure time for developing intimacy and enjoying sensual moments. Stay open-minded—the very anticipation of no longer enjoying sex can limit your options.

Some women do report a decline in sexual desire at menopause, but about one-third of all women report no noticeable change. Male sex hormones or androgens such as testosterone, rather than the female sex hormone estrogen, are associated with libido. While androgen production does decline with menopause, many other body tissues take over the production of androgens once production by the ovaries declines. Androgens are produced in skin tissue, body fat, brain tissue, muscles, the pineal gland, and even hair follicles. In addition, many other factors play a role in maintaining sexual drive, including diet and general energy level and state of health.

Menopausal symptoms such as hot flashes and night sweats can take so much energy that little is left for sex. A woman may experience skin sensitivity. In addition, there is a natural thinning of vaginal tissues and reduced production of lubricating fluids that normally facilitate intercourse. However, there are many exceptions, especially if women remain sexually active and if they have sufficient body fat to help maintain estrogen levels.

How the Body Changes

As ovarian function wanes, blood flow to the pelvic area declines. In the areas of the vagina and vulva (the outer portion of the female genitalia), this decrease can be as much as 60%. Pubic hair also thins and becomes coarser.

The most pronounced changes occur to the vagina. Vaginal tissue is made up of many layers of cushioning cells. When the supply of estrogen is adequate, these cells remain resilient and strong. However, with menopause, the outer layers of vaginal mucosal cells, approximately six layers deep, can become thin. The inner surface of the vagina begins to flatten and loses its rough, ridged appearance. The vagina also decreases in depth and the walls of the vagina begin to lose their elasticity as fibrous connective tissue replaces muscle cells. However, orgasmic contractions of the vagina still occur after menopause.

Another result of diminished blood flow is that production of vaginal fluid begins to fluctuate and is less copious. A lack of lubricating fluid can cause intercourse to be somewhat painful and irritating to vaginal tissue. If this tissue has thinned, sexual activity can be all the more irritating to the vaginal walls. Fortunately, many treatments and behavior changes have been shown to alleviate these conditions. These are covered in Chapters 4 through 9.

Vaginitis

Postmenopausal women are more likely to develop vaginitis, inflammation of the vagina. The most common form is *atrophic vaginitis*, since it is related to the thinning of vaginal tissue.

Symptoms include itching or burning and a thin, watery discharge that occasionally may be tinged with blood. (If you notice blood, have this assessed by a physician to rule out the presence of cancer.) The vagina may also be more susceptible to infections. One study of 821 women found that vaginal infections were six times more common than urinary tract infections. Vaginitis is one of the most common reasons menopausal women seek medical attention.

A balanced diet, low in refined foods, sugars, and fats, is generally recommended for vaginitis. Useful nutrients include zinc, vitamin A, vitamin C, vitamin E, manganese, and B complex. In particular, live-culture yogurt has been shown to prevent vaginitis. Replenishing the vagina with desirable bacteria helps reverse this condition. In a 1992 study published in the *Annals of Internal Medicine*, researchers worked with 33 women who were troubled by recurrent vaginitis caused by infection with candida. The women added live-culture yogurt to their diet for 6 months. At the end of the trial period, this group of women were three times less likely to develop vaginitis than they had been before yogurt was added to their meals.

The brand of yogurt you buy must contain live lactobacillus cultures. Only buy products that state this on the label, and avoid yogurt products that include fruit and added sugars. Stick with plain yogurt.

Symptoms versus Disease

The problems described in this chapter are not the only complaints associated with menopause. Medical problems such as osteoporosis and heart disease, as well as ailments such as incontinence and thyroid problems, are often presented as symptoms. But strictly speaking, these are degenerative diseases, the consequences of lifestyle. You may be at higher risk for these after menopause, but it is important to keep separate in your mind the subject of menopause and these undesirable and even frightening conditions. Menopause is not about illness and declining function. Menopause is a natural life event. You can skip ahead to Chapter 10 if you want to know more about various ailments that become more common as women age. Learn all you can about their causes and how to take care of yourself to prevent them, but as you read, remember that menopause has not sentenced you to these problems.

CHAPTER THREE

Creating a Healthy and Empowering Passage through Menopause: Getting Started on the Six-Step Healthy Menopause Program

Now that you've been introduced to some of the prevailing attitudes toward menopause, as well as the symptoms of menopause and their origins, you are ready to begin shaping your own passage through the change. The following chapters give you many tools, ranging from natural therapies to hormone replacement therapy. You'll find out about traditional remedies gathered over centuries as well as current research on menopause. The Healthy Menopause Program takes you through this wealth of information in six easy steps. If you follow this plan, you can look forward to:

- Having solutions at your fingertips for lessening and even preventing menopause symptoms
- Being better able to manage stress and feeling more relaxed

- Lowering your risk of degenerative diseases such as osteoporosis and heart disease
- Enjoying a healthy and empowering attitude toward menopause
- Having a sense of vitality and well-being

But where do you begin? How do you pick and choose among all the information and tailor a plan of action suited to your own individual needs? Begin by keeping a record of how you feel. Start a menopause journal.

Your Menopause Journal

You need to develop a way of keeping a record of your menopausal symptoms that works for you. If you are always on the run, carrying a small notebook in your purse may be the only way you can be sure to write down when symptoms occur. Use a page for each day. You can accumulate useful information this way, especially if you also write down what you've been eating or if you have had difficulty sleeping—factors that can trigger symptoms. However, thumbing through pages makes it difficult to have an overview of how you've been feeling or to decipher possible reasons why. For this reason, even if you begin with just a notebook, you will probably soon decide to keep your notes in a calendar format.

Choose a page size and format that suits the amount of information you plan to write down. Stationery and office-supply stores sell month-at-a-glance and week-at-a-glance calendars. Keep this calendar where you are likely to remember to write in it, for instance, in a frequently used desk drawer at work or on a nightstand next to your bed.

Using a calendar as a menopause diary allows you to easily see changes in symptoms and the patterns in which they occur. A month-at-a-glance calendar is an ideal format for tracking the regularity of the menstrual cycle during perimenopause when timing begins to become erratic. Using a calendar can also help you spot a sequence of events that ultimately trigger a symptom. What you write down can help you identify associations, leading you to write down events that you might have otherwise overlooked. For instance, you may have noticed a link between hot flashes, anxiety, and being caught in commuter traffic. Then your journal may need to include traffic data. Your own story will begin to show up in your notes as the weeks pass—a sign that you're doing a great job journaling!

You may even want to work with a daily calendar that is divided into hours for more detailed record keeping. This format allows you to easily jot down what you eat, when you eat it, the hour of the day you usually feel tired, and other daily habits and experiences.

Be a Sleuth

Noticing an association between symptoms and activities and events can give you clues about treating menopausal problems. For instance, let's say you note that you routinely have breakfast at 8:00 A.M., lunch at noon, and dinner at 6:00 P.M., and you regularly write that your anxiety increases around 11:30 A.M. and between 4 and 5 P.M. each day. Such detailed journaling can give you an important piece of information—that your anxiety is brought on by a lack of fuel reaching your brain, a well-known phenomenon, because you haven't eaten for several hours. And now you have a solution—having a nutritious snack between meals. As you use your journal, it can become an increasingly valuable tool for managing your menopause. No one but you can gather such important information.

Charting Symptoms

If you don't particularly like writing in a diary, you can use a simpler format for keeping menopause records. Chart your symptoms or whatever data you want to follow. Then all you'll need to do is make a check in a box. The number of checks will quickly give you a picture of whatever information you are recording.

Set up your own chart on a piece of graph paper. Across the top of the page, write the days of the week. Then, to keep a record of frequency of symptoms, write a list of symptoms down the left-hand side of the page. This format is shown on the following page.

Then take a ruler and draw lines down the page and across so that for each day there is a box that refers to symptoms. Use the graph paper lines as your guide. When a symptom occurs, simply make a check in that box. Three hot flashes on Tuesday results in three checks in the Tuesday hot-flash box.

Along with this chart, you might also make a second, with days of the week across the top and an informal list of symptom triggers listed down the left-hand margin. You can use the two charts together, for any given day of the week, to look for an association between symptoms and behavior. A sample chart follows on page 40.

Working with the Six-Step Healthy Menopause Program

Journaling can work hand-in-hand with the six-step program for menopause. Refer back and forth between this text and your journal to figure out what changes you need to make in the way you live and what treatments you may need. The Six-Step Healthy Menopause Program gives you six powerful ways of ensuring your health as a woman. Here's a quick overview of each approach.

Step 1: Nutrients and Menopause
A wide range of vitamins and minerals play a vital role in supporting female health, and some are particularly important for

Symptom Frequency Chart

Symptom	Monday	Tuesday	Wednesday	Thursday	Friday	Saturday	Sunday
Hot flashes							
Fatigue							
Mood swings							
Anxiety							
Irritability							
Depression							
Poor memory							
Vaginal dryness							
Lack of sex drive							

Symptom Trigger Chart

Trigger	Monday	Tuesday	Wednesday	Thursday	Friday	Saturday	Sunday
Ate refined sugar							
Drank cola							
Had coffee							
Ate red meat							
Skipped supplements							
No exercise							
Lots of stress							

menopause. For instance, vitamin E is considered a prime menopausal nutrient, as it nourishes the reproductive system. Many other vitamins and major and trace minerals are also essential. In Step 1, you will learn about the foods that are excellent sources of certain nutrients and find out about the benefits of taking nutrient supplements to make up for certain deficiencies.

Phytoestrogens are a special category of nutrients that have been studied extensively in recent years. Menopausal symptoms can be brought on by hormone imbalances, which can be corrected with phytoestrogens. Bioflavonoids and boron, two relatively unfamiliar nutrients, also bolster female health. These compounds are subtle but powerful tools for maintaining health as you pass through menopause.

Step 2: Diet and Menopause

Good health at menopause begins with eating quality foods. Step 2 tells you all about the many natural, unprocessed, and unrefined whole foods that women need. These foods are especially rich in nutrients that support hormonal balance and nourish various body systems. There may be some surprises for you on the list of recommended foods. New research shows that butter is better for you than margarine, and certain essential oils are required eating! Fruits, vegetables, legumes, nuts, and seeds are high on the list, and fish is another best bet. Healthy meals are made with savory, sweet, spicy ingredients that are full of color and taste appeal.

Foods to avoid are also covered. These are the energy and health depleters—white sugar, white flour, colas, coffee, and overly processed and fast foods of all sorts. A woman subsisting on such fare during the years leading up to menopause may enter this transition deficient in certain vitamins and minerals. This can translate into annoying menopausal symptoms and poor health later in life. Step 2 turns you into a health-wise consumer of nature's best foods.

Step 3: Herbs and Menopause

A close cousin to eating well for menopause is using herbs to treat symptoms and reverse them. Some herbs such as black cohosh and dong quai help balance hormones. Others like chamomile are ideal for their calming effects. The range of plant substances used medicinally to treat menopause has evolved over centuries, as women have experimented with one herb and then another. In addition, many herbs have recently been put to the test in scientific studies. Today, their properties and actions are well known. If you are looking for a safe and reliable way of treating menopausal symptoms, Step 3 is a good place to start.

Step 4: Exercise and Menopause

This step of the Six-Step Healthy Menopause Program is not optional! You cannot expect to have good health and not move your body. Step 4 introduces you to the types of pleasurable physical exercise that have been proven to reduce certain menopausal symptoms, as well as promote long-term health.

Yoga, tai chi, and chi gong are soothing and relaxing and also stimulate the system. Every woman passing through menopause can benefit from these gentle forms of exercise. But vigorous exercise also has its benefits. A good workout that results in shedding a little perspiration energizes the system, speeds elimination of toxins, dispels angst, and helps keep the heart healthy. Weight-bearing exercise, which includes lifting weights and walking, is especially good for women, as this activity strengthens bones. Add Step 4 to your life and you'll benefit in many ways. Sports, dance, and physical challenges add richness to life.

Step 5: Stress Management and Menopause

Stress, both physical and emotional, is a well-known trigger of menopausal symptoms. For instance, hot flashes and everyday annoyances often go hand in hand. Step 5 tells you about how the body's reaction to stress can affect crucial aspects of female health such as hormone production. The adrenal glands, which secrete hormones that govern the stress response, also are involved in the production of a significant amount of estrogen postmenopause. The syntheses of both types of hormones are closely related, and when stress places demands on adrenal function, estrogen output declines.

This valuable step introduces you to the various vitamins and minerals that are depleted by stress. Certain foods replenish these while others deplete reserves. Herbs and exercise are useful tools in managing the stress response. Step 5 explains how to relax by using paced breathing and quiet time to meditate. Experiment with these approaches and find a mix that works for you.

Step 6: Hormone Replacement Therapy

Many problems associated with menopause are due to an imbalance of hormones and to reduced production of hormones. The most direct way to address these changes is by supplementing with the missing hormones, such as estrogen and progesterone. Of course, you'll need to consult with a physician who can test for your current levels of hormone production and give you a prescription for the specific hormones and dosages you need.

Supplemental hormones are available in many forms, including pills, patches, and creams. The most widely used are synthetic and have a chemical structure different from that which the female body produces. But these days, "natural" hormones are also available, in particular through independent, compounding pharmacies, which customize hormonal therapies based on individual patient's needs. These hormones have the same structure as the body's hormones and often cause fewer side effects. Step 6 helps you sort your way through the products and options to decide if supplemental hormones are for you. Whatever your decision, remember that Step 6 cannot replace Steps 1 through 5.

Check In with Yourself

The following chapters give you the Six-Step Healthy Menopause Program in depth. You are guaranteed to be exposed to lots of useful information. Of course, this will do you no good if you don't make use of it. Before you begin reading more, stop a moment and ask yourself how likely you'll be to follow the advice. Your compliance is an essential part of the Healthy Menopause Program! We all have our excuses. Not enough time, not enough money, and so on. A lifetime habit of putting your needs second to others can also keep you from starting this program.

Indeed, accomplishing what you say you'd like to do can be difficult, as life is so busy and complex. Circumstances can prevent you from following the Healthy Menopause Program as you might like, but being aware of the usual excuses may help you keep to your plan.

For starters, make a list of your favorite excuses. How can I think about menopause when I am so busy at work? I'm just too tired to start changing what I eat or figuring out new ways to take care of myself. The thought of menopause makes me feel old and I rather not think about it. And so on. What reasons do you fall back on, time and again—reasons that seem very real to you? If you hold on to your goal of excellent health passionately enough, you can get past these. In fact, you can use menopause to banish your old reliable excuses from the rest of your life as well. Think of how freeing that would be!

Most of the recommendations in this program require little additional time or money. Eating nutritious foods doesn't have to cost more. Being better able to manage stress can actually save you time and energy. If you are worried about feeling overburdened by beginning the program, look for simple ways to begin to incorporate the various steps of this program into your life. One change can lead to another. The sooner you start, the sooner you'll benefit.

CHAPTER FOUR

Step 1: Nutrients and Menopause— Vitamins, Minerals, and Special Nutrients

Sufficient intake of vitamins, minerals, and special nutrients is an integral part of the Six-Step Healthy Menopause Program. This chapter tells you all about them and explains the many functions they perform in terms of menopause. Phyto-estrogens and essential fatty acids are especially featured.

Nutrients are workhorses, required components of hundreds of chemical reactions that are continuously taking place within body cells and supporting life. When your body sends signals that it is hungry, nutrients are what it is asking for, not just calories. Browse through the following information on vitamins, minerals, and special nutrients to have a sense of just how important each one is for female health. And for an overview, take a look at the section at the end of this chapter that lists various menopausal symptoms and the nutrients that are most effective for treating them.

Food Sources of Nutrients
Versus Supplements

If you are barely troubled by menopause and eat a balanced diet, you may be able to consume sufficient amounts of nutrients through the everyday foods you eat. However, most individuals would benefit from also taking vitamin and mineral supplements. You can't always trust food to supply you with what it's supposed to contain. If produce is grown on land depleted of minerals, the mineral content of the food will also be lower. Transporting, processing, and storing foods also destroys the nutritional value of many food products. And if you are troubled by menopausal symptoms, which can be a sign of nutrient deficiencies, you will most likely need to take supplements in therapeutic dosages. You could never eat enough food to consume the higher quantities of nutrients that are required for treating certain symptoms. You'll find a list of suggested nutrients and the amounts to take later in this chapter.

Vitamins

Without vitamins, your body would not be able to function. Having sufficient levels of vitamins, as well as enzymes, speeds the making or breaking of chemical bonds that join molecules together. These reactions drive cellular activity and make the production of energy possible. If you reach menopause low on vitamins, deficiency symptoms such as fatigue and irritability can show up—problems blamed on menopause that simply may be the result of poor eating habits.

The information in this chapter tells you what foods are particularly high in the various vitamins. If you rarely eat many of these foods, start adding them to your grocery list. A word of warning about cooking such foods: Vitamins have a chemistry that is more delicate and unstable than minerals. Since vitamins can be readily destroyed in cooking, each of the following sections concludes with tips on cooking foods to preserve these fragile nutrients.

Vitamin A and Beta-Carotene

Vitamin A, a fat-soluble vitamin, is found in meats and other animal foods, while the *carotenoids*, a family of water-soluble vitamins that have vitamin A activity, are supplied by plant foods. One type of carotenoid, beta-carotene, is well known, but there are actually over 400 different carotenoids, each important for health in their own way.

Carotenoids are actually red and yellow pigments—the coloring agents that give red peppers, carrots, and golden acorn squash their hue. All green vegetables also contain beta-carotene, but the pigment can't be seen because the green chlorophyll masks it.

BENEFITS

- Vitamin A is important for skin growth and repair, thereby helping to maintain moist outer skin and inner vaginal tissue.

- Vitamin A helps slow physical changes that begin to show up postmenopause.

- Beginning at midlife, a woman's night vision may begin to decline, making such activities as night driving much more difficult. Night vision depends upon having adequate stores of vitamin A. The vitamin A you consume, through a series of chemical reactions, becomes part of the photoreceptor cells in the eye that make it possible for you to differentiate between light and dark.

- With age, hair may lack luster, which is also a sign of vitamin A deficiency.

- Vitamin A stimulates the immune system, and beta-carotene in particular acts as an antioxidant, destroying free radicals that can lead to cancer.

BEST FOOD SOURCES OF VITAMIN A

Vegetables: sweet potatoes, carrots, butternut squash, spinach

Fruit: cantaloupe, mango, apricot

Meats: beef and calf's liver (preferably organic)

Dairy: butter (preferably organic)

Miscellaneous: eggs

COOKING TIPS

- To preserve fat-soluble vitamin A in meats, avoid cooking them at very high temperatures. Frying meats damages their vitamin A by oxidizing it. Sauté meats and roast at lower temperatures for a longer time instead.

- To maximize your intake of the carotenes, cook carotene-containing vegetables so that the cell walls break down and release the vitamins, which are then easier to absorb. Steam or bake carrots and yellow squash, excellent sources of this vitamin, and better yet, serve these vegetables puréed or mashed. This method of preparation turns familiar foods into new and interesting dishes.

B-Complex Vitamins

There are 11 B-complex vitamins. The most well known are thiamin (B_1), riboflavin (B_2), niacin (B_3), pantothenic acid (B_5), vitamin B_6 (pyridoxine), B_{12} (cobalamin), and folic acid. The remaining four are choline, inositol, biotin, and para-aminobenzoic acid (PABA). These latter four are present in liver, eggs, unprocessed whole grains, and molasses.

The complete complex of B vitamins works together to nourish the nervous system and stabilize brain chemistry. These vitamins are essential for the conversion of food into energy, and help maintain healthy skin and hair. Stress uses up B vitamins, which can become depleted by such body changes as menopause.

Thiamin, B_1

BENEFITS

- Thiamin supports the health of the nervous system. A deficiency of B_1 can result in irritability.
- Thiamin helps keep the mind sharp. A lack of vitamin B_1 is associated with an inability to concentrate, as well as memory loss, which can occur during menopause.

BEST FOOD SOURCES OF THIAMIN

Whole grains: rye, rice, wheat, millet, buckwheat, bulgur

Beans: pinto, black, garbanzo, soy, black-eyed peas

Vegetables: potatoes, peas, Jerusalem artichokes, corn, okra

Fruit: watermelon, avocado

Nuts: Brazil nuts, pine nuts, pistachios

Seeds: sunflower seeds

Meats: pork, liver, quail

Fish: lobster, trout, oysters

COOKING TIPS

Thiamin is the second least stable vitamin, after vitamin C. Because it is water soluble, chopped and minced vegetables can lose up to 70% of this vitamin in the cooking liquid—a good reason to save the juice for soups. Cook potatoes in their jackets. Thiamin is stable in acidic-based foods but not in alkaline-based foods, so baking powder in baked goods can cut by half the amount of thiamin present in flour. The thiamin in meats, fish, and poultry is best preserved by roasting, broiling, and braising, and is reduced by stewing and frying.

Riboflavin, B$_2$

BENEFITS

- Strengthens adrenal function, thereby supporting hormone balance and lessening susceptibility to menopausal symptoms
- Generally slows the aging process by helping maintain good vision, healthy hair and nails, and youthful skin, including vaginal tissue
- Helps sustain energy by increasing the ability of the cells to use oxygen

BEST FOOD SOURCES OF RIBOFLAVIN

Whole grains: wild rice, millet, wheat

Fish: clams, salmon, mackerel, trout, herring

Vegetables: yams, mushrooms, winter squash

Fruit: avocado

Beans: pinto, black

Meat: liver (preferably organic), dark-meat chicken

Nuts: almonds, hazelnuts, chestnuts, cashews

Seeds: pumpkin

Dairy: milk, yogurt

COOKING TIPS

- Light is the greatest destroyer of riboflavin, but this is not usually a problem since milk products and bread are usually stored in the dark. Nuts and seeds should also be stored away from light.

- Riboflavin is diminished when food is chopped and cooked, especially when the food is cooked in a lot of liquid, since riboflavin is water soluble. Steam or bake instead. Enjoy some riboflavin-rich foods raw and whole.

Niacin, B_3

BENEFITS

- Helps stabilize blood sugar, which when fluctuating dramatically, can trigger a range of menopausal symptoms
- Supports mental clarity and memory, since niacin plays a role in brain metabolism
- Increases energy by improving circulation
- Sustains sexual function by benefiting vaginal tissue and stimulating the formation of mucus in response to sexual activity
- Lowers cholesterol

BEST FOOD SOURCES OF NIACIN

Meat: liver, beef, chicken, turkey

Fish: tuna, salmon, halibut, oysters, shrimp, sardines

Vegetables: mushrooms, potatoes, asparagus, broccoli, summer squash

Fruit: peaches, cantaloupe

Nuts: peanuts

Whole grains: whole wheat, corn tortillas (To make corn tortillas, Mexicans soak their maize in lime water overnight in order to free the niacin in the grain from its inactive bound form.)

COOKING TIPS

- Niacin is very stable. Cooking a food containing niacin makes the vitamin easier to absorb.

- When you cook meat, water-soluble niacin accumulates in the meat juices. By making a sauce from the juices, you can add the niacin back into the dish you are preparing.

Pantothenic Acid, B₅

BENEFITS

- Essential for optimal adrenal function and necessary for hormonal health postmenopause
- Helps in the management of stress by increasing the production of the adrenal hormone, cortisone, thereby reducing the frequency and severity of menopausal symptoms
- Necessary for proper brain function
- Aids in the prevention of premature aging and wrinkling of the skin

BEST FOOD SOURCES OF PANTOTHENIC ACID

Meat: beef liver (preferably organic), chicken

Fish: blue fish, abalone, trout, salmon, cod

Fruit: avocado, pomegranate

COOKING TIPS

- Raw foods are the best source. Pantothenic acid is easily destroyed in cooking if heat is coupled with ingredients that are especially acidic or alkalinic, such as vinegar or baking soda.
- The low temperatures used in deep freezing can destroy pantothenic acid. However, pantothenic acid's presence in such a wide variety of foods may compensate for its fragility.

Pyridoxine, B_6

BENEFITS

- Combats both depression and stress through its interaction with amino acids in the brain and adrenal hormones
- Strengthens collagen, the structural component of skin tissue, supporting a more youthful appearance
- Lessens edema and leg cramps that can occur during perimenopause

BEST FOOD SOURCES OF PYRIDOXINE

Meat: liver (preferably organic), beef, pork, turkey, chicken

Fish: trout, salmon, bluefish

Whole grains: brown rice, wheat, rye, bulgur wheat

Nuts: walnuts, hazelnuts, peanuts, chestnuts

Seeds: sunflower

Beans: pinto, navy, lima

Fruit: mango, banana, avocado, plantain, melon

Miscellaneous: blackstrap molasses

COOKING TIPS

- B_6 is not affected significantly by heat and air, and is very stable in the presence of acidic and alkalinic substances.
- This water-soluble vitamin can be lost when food is overcooked. After cooking meats and fish, be sure to serve these foods with the pan juices, which contain some of this vitamin.

Cobalamin, B_{12}

BENEFITS

- Maintains memory and mental clarity
- Promotes energy

BEST FOOD SOURCES OF COBALAMIN

Meat: liver, beef, pork, lamb

Fish: clams, oysters, herring, eel, snails, trout

Dairy: yogurt

Miscellaneous: eggs

COOKING TIPS

- Use dry cooking methods such as baking to prevent B_{12} from leaking into cooking liquids. However, if you eat animal foods, you are not likely to be deficient, as they are excellent sources of this nutrient. In addition, the body normally stores a 5- to 6-year supply.

- Vitamin B_{12} is unstable when exposed to alkaline substances, such as baking soda, but is stable in all other foods.

Folic Acid

BENEFITS

- Lessens irritability
- Promotes mental clarity and memory
- Helps prevent fatigue

BEST FOOD SOURCES OF FOLIC ACID

Vegetables: asparagus, beets, turnip greens, peas, artichokes, okra, leeks

Fruit: avocado, boysenberries, cantaloupe, oranges, loganberries, strawberries

Fish: trout, oysters, tuna

Meat: liver (preferably organic), beef, pork, lamb

Poultry: turkey, chicken, quail

Whole grains: whole wheat, barley, brown rice

Nuts: pistachios

Beans: soy

COOKING TIPS

- Folic acid can leak out during cooking. Steam vegetables, and when cooking meats, use the juices to make a sauce.

- This B vitamin is susceptible to high temperatures and light, and can be lost when food is left at room temperature for a long period of time. Be sure to refrigerate vegetables and store grains in opaque containers in a cool place.

Vitamin C

BENEFITS

- Essential for the formation of the hormone, adrenaline, produced by the adrenal glands to manage stress, which can worsen symptoms of menopause

- May help prevent hot flashes when coupled with vitamin E

- Helps maintain skin quality and mucous membranes in the vagina in its role in the formation of collagen, a part of the connective tissue in skin and ligaments

- Creates a mildly acidic environment in the stomach, which increases the amount of calcium that a woman can absorb, helping to prevent weakening of the bones

- Functions as a powerful antioxidant to slow aging and reduce the risk of heart disease and possibly cancer

BEST FOOD SOURCES OF VITAMIN C

Vegetables: sweet peppers, broccoli, brussels sprouts, kale, lamb's-quarter, alfalfa sprouts, tomatoes

Fruit: papaya, quava, kiwi, citrus, cantaloupe, strawberries, acerola cherries, black currants

Tea: rose hips

COOKING TIPS

- Vitamin C is the least stable vitamin and can be lost when exposed to light, heat, or air. A freshly sliced orange, rather than juice, is a good source of this vitamin.

- Steaming vegetables preserves more of their vitamin C than boiling them.

- Vitamin C is highest in raw vegetables.

Vitamin D

BENEFITS

- Essential for the absorption of calcium, which helps maintain proper skeletal composition and bone strength

- Supports the health of the nervous system

- Helps maintain normal heart action and normal clotting of the blood

- Treats dry skin when applied as an ointment, along with vitamin A and zinc

BEST FOOD SOURCES OF VITAMIN D

Fish: kippers, mackerel, salmon, sardines, herring, halibut

Meat: liver (preferably organic)

Miscellaneous: egg yolk, sunshine

COOKING TIPS

- Vitamin D is very stable and remains in fish even when smoked.

Vitamin E (Tocopherol)

BENEFITS

- Effectively reduces hot flashes in about 40% of cases
- Recommended for tempering anxiety associated with menopause
- Helps lessen menopausal fatigue caused by lack of sleep due to night sweats
- Maintains moist skin and healthy vaginal tissue
- Functions as an antioxidant to help prevent heart disease and slow the aging process

BEST FOOD SOURCES OF VITAMIN E

Cold-pressed, unrefined oils: safflower, sesame, peanut, soy, wheat germ

Whole grains: millet, oatmeal, wheat, corn

Nuts: almonds, Brazil nuts, hazelnuts, peanuts

Seeds: sunflower

Vegetables: sweet potatoes, asparagus, cucumber, kale, collards, seaweed

Beans: navy

Fish: haddock, mackerel, herring, salmon

Meat: lamb, organ meats

Fruit: mango

Miscellaneous: eggs, molasses

COOKING TIPS

- Vitamin E is very sensitive to oxidation, particularly in the presence of heat and alkaline-based foods.
- Enjoy fresh (not frozen) foods, whole grains, and unrefined oils, which have higher levels of vitamin E than their more refined and processed counterparts.

Minerals

Your system also requires minerals as components of body enzymes that catalyze vital chemical reactions within body tissues. Minerals are essential for healthy bones, the proper composition of the blood, and the maintenance of normal cell function. Having an adequate intake can help ensure your health and well-being during and postmenopause.

You are likely to have some mineral deficiencies if you eat a lot of refined and processed foods. In addition, minerals are not as readily absorbed as vitamins. They compete with each other for absorption. Once absorbed, they can bind with other substances and may then be excreted before they are put to work. To ensure an adequate supply, include plenty of mineral-rich foods in every meal.

COOKING TIPS FOR PRESERVING MINERALS
Minerals are chemically far more stable than vitamins. The same cooking pointers apply to all minerals:

- Wash vegetables such as leafy greens and then chop them for cooking. If you chop before washing, minerals are released into the washing water.

- Avoid overcooking vegetables to the extent that cell walls rupture, releasing minerals into the cooking liquid.

- If you like eating your vegetables well cooked and very tender, make sure to save the cooking liquid. Sip it as a broth or add it to soup.

- Steam vegetables or bake them; do not boil them.

- When cooking meat, remember to deglaze the pan and make a sauce of the mineral-rich meat juices. To deglaze, simply heat a small amount of wine or stock in the pan and stir to loosen any browned bits of food on the bottom.

Boron

BENEFITS

- Helps reduce loss of calcium from bones
- May be necessary for the synthesis of estrogen
- Enhances the effects of supplemental estrogen

BEST FOOD SOURCES OF BORON

Fruit: apples, pears, peaches, grapes, raisins, dates

Vegetables: dark leafy greens, potatoes, broccoli, parsley

Nuts: almonds, hazelnuts, peanuts

Beans: soy

Beverages: wine, cider, beer

Miscellaneous: honey, cinnamon

Boron is making a comeback. Once a food preservative, in the form of boric acid, and then retired from that role, it is now being studied for its importance in various aspects of female health. Though the mechanisms are still unclear, it is thought to function at the cellular level to affect various systems. A deficiency of boron can negatively affect calcium metabolism, motor skills, and mental alertness. It also appears to enhance the effectiveness of supplemental estrogen. Although the presence of boron is negligible in animal foods, it can be found in many plant foods.

Calcium

BENEFITS

- Contributes to bone structure and strength
- Helps prevent nervousness, irritability, headaches, and insomnia and is crucial to the flow of impulses along nerves
- Maintains muscle tone and elasticity and helps prevent leg cramps

- Regulates the heartbeat, helping to prevent the heart palpitations sometimes associated with menopause
- Contributes to maintenance of normal blood pressure and blood lipids

BEST FOOD SOURCES OF CALCIUM

Dairy products: milk, cheese, plain yogurt

Vegetables: turnip greens, bok choy, collards, mustard greens, kale, cabbage, kelp, okra

Fruit: figs, cherimoyas, papayas, oranges, boysenberries

Fish: canned sardines, mackerel, and salmon with bones; shrimp

Nuts: hazelnuts, Brazil nuts, almonds

Seeds: sesame

Beans: soy, kidney, pinto, chickpeas, Great Northern

Whole grains: cornmeal, whole wheat, brown rice, bulgur

Miscellaneous: blackstrap molasses

Chromium

BENEFITS

- Helps stabilize blood sugar levels, thus reducing a variety of menopausal symptoms
- May help ensure heart health

BEST FOOD SOURCES OF CHROMIUM

Vegetables: mushrooms, beets, asparagus, seaweed, potatoes

Fruit: prunes, grapes

Meats: liver (preferably organic), beef

Poultry: turkey

Whole grains: whole wheat, brown rice

Beverages: wine, beer, maple syrup

Miscellaneous: wheat germ, brewer's yeast, honey

Though chromium deficiency is rare in other countries, in North America it is very common. When foods are refined, chromium is often removed. In addition, diets high in sugar have been shown to increase the excretion of chromium.

Copper

BENEFITS

- Necessary for the formation of collagen, which gives structure to bones and skin
- Contributes to the mineral content of bones
- Aids in the formation of pigment in the skin and hair, contributing to a more youthful appearance
- Helps maintain the health of the nervous system

BEST FOOD SOURCES OF COPPER

Beans: soy, chickpeas, navy, kidney, lentils, black-eyed peas, Great Northern

Nuts: cashews, Brazil nuts, hazelnuts, pistachio, walnuts

Seeds: sunflower, sesame

Meat: liver (preferably organic)

Seafood: oysters, squid, mussels, clams, crab

Vegetables: potatoes

Fruit: avocado

Miscellaneous: molasses

Supplementing with zinc can lower a woman's reserves of copper. Zinc can interfere with the absorption and utilization of copper; these minerals must be kept in balance.

Iodine

BENEFITS

- Maintains energy through its role in thyroid function
- Helps prevent hypothyroidism, a condition in which secretion of thyroid hormone is diminished and consequently metabolism slows, which is more common postmenopause
- Promotes mental and physical alertness
- Maintains healthy hair, nails, skin, and teeth
- Helps prevent hardening of the arteries

BEST FOOD SOURCES OF IODINE

Fish: haddock, perch, salmon, tuna, sole, oysters, shrimp

Poultry: eggs

Meat: liver (preferably organic)

Vegetables: spinach, potatoes, broccoli, mushrooms, asparagus

Dairy: plain yogurt

Miscellaneous: eggs

Iron

BENEFITS

- Maintains energy by facilitating the transport of oxygen to the cells
- Helps retain a rosy pallor

BEST FOOD SOURCES OF IRON

Meat: liver and other organ meats, beef, pork, lamb

Fish: clams, oysters, tuna, abalone, shrimp, caviar

Whole grains: millet, rice, wild rice, buckwheat, whole wheat

Beans: black, navy, chickpeas, soy, kidney, lima

Vegetables: artichokes, parsley, leeks, peas, green onions, spinach, beets

Fruit: raisins, peaches, figs, currants, boysenberries, prunes

Nuts: almonds, cashews, Brazil nuts, hazelnuts

Miscellaneous: eggs

During perimenopause, menstrual flow can become heavy, resulting in a loss of iron-rich blood. Iron can also be lost in perspiration.

The iron in meat is most easily absorbed, whereas the iron in vegetables, which is in another chemical form, is better absorbed in the presence of vitamin C. Our bodies absorb only about 10% of all the iron we eat.

Note: Supplementing with iron is not recommended as freely as it once was because recent studies have suggested that excess stores of iron may increase the risk of heart disease and cancer. Make food your source.

Magnesium

BENEFITS

- May reduce the frequency and severity of hot flashes in some women
- Counteracts menopausal fatigue and muscle weakness
- Helps prevent irritability and depression associated with menopause
- Plays a role in stabilizing blood sugar levels, which can affect symptoms

- Prevents irregular or rapid heartbeat due to deficiency
- Essential for long-term health of the nervous system, heart, and skeletal system, helping to prevent related diseases of aging

BEST FOOD SOURCES OF MAGNESIUM

Vegetables: spinach, kale, beet greens, broccoli, potatoes with their skins

Grains: buckwheat, whole wheat, cornmeal, bulgur, whole rye, millet, brown rice

Beans: soy, lima, Great Northern, chickpeas, black, pinto, kidney, navy

Fruit: figs, plantains, avocados

Nuts: cashews, Brazil nuts, walnuts, almonds, pine nuts, hazelnuts

Seeds: pumpkin, squash, watermelon, sesame, sunflower, flax

Fish: shrimp, oysters, halibut, mackerel

Miscellaneous: egg yolks, blackstrap molasses, chocolate, tahini, tofu

Manganese

BENEFITS

- Helps maintain the production of sex hormones in its role as catalyst for the formation of cholesterol from which estrogen is made
- Nourishes the nervous system and brain
- Plays a role in the functioning of the adrenal glands, which secrete hormones that prepare the body to withstand stress
- Supports normal thyroid function

- Essential for bone growth and development as well as heart health

BEST FOOD SOURCES OF MANGANESE

Fish: clams, bass, trout, pike, perch, smelts, oysters

Grains: whole wheat, brown rice, buckwheat

Beans: lima, chickpeas, soy, navy, lentils, pinto, Great Northern, kidney, black-eyed peas

Vegetables: collards, okra, peas, seaweed

Fruit: pineapple, banana, blackberries, raspberries, grapes, blueberries

Nuts: Brazil, chestnuts, hazelnuts, almonds, peanuts

Seeds: sunflower

Miscellaneous: chocolate, carob, black tea

Phosphorus

BENEFITS

- Necessary for the transport of calcium to the bones, helping to prevent osteoporosis
- Important for the regular contractions of the heart, helping to prevent heart palpitations
- Supports healthy nerves and mental function

BEST FOOD SOURCES OF PHOSPHORUS

Fish: mackerel, lobster, bluefish, crab, catfish, salmon, flounder

Whole grains: brown rice, cornmeal, wheat, oats, rye, quinoa

Beans: chickpeas, soy

Fruit: peaches, apricots, raisins, figs, prunes

Nuts: Brazil nuts, peanuts, almonds, cashews, pistachios, walnuts

Seeds: pumpkin, sunflower, sesame

Meat: pork, beef, liver

Poultry: chicken, turkey, duck

Dairy: butter, cheese

Miscellaneous: brewer's yeast, eggs

Potassium

BENEFITS

- Essential for avoiding irritability, nervousness, and fatigue
- Helps regulate thyroid function, which maintains energy production
- Plays a role in the stress response, which can affect menopausal symptoms
- Helps normalize heartbeat and stabilize blood pressure

BEST FOOD SOURCES OF POTASSIUM

Meat: beef, pork, lamb

Fish: cod, flounder, trout, halibut

Vegetables: potatoes, Swiss chard

Fruit: raisins, papaya, plantain, figs, currants, cantaloupe, apricots, banana, avocado

Beans: white, lima, soy, black, kidney, split peas, lentils

Nuts: pistachios, almonds, peanuts, Brazil nuts

Seeds: sunflower, sesame

Whole grains: rye, millet, buckwheat, barley

Selenium

BENEFITS

- Works with vitamin E to reduce symptoms of menopause such as hot flashes

- Preserves tissue elasticity and helps maintain vaginal lubrication

- As an antioxidant, lowers risk of heart disease and some cancers

BEST FOOD SOURCES OF SELENIUM

Nuts: Brazil nuts

Seeds: sesame

Meat: liver (preferably organic), beef, lamb, kidney

Poultry: chicken

Fish: shrimp, smelts, clams, lobsters, scallops, cod, flat fish, tuna

Whole grains: whole wheat, brown rice

Vegetables: carrots, cabbage, mushrooms, corn, potatoes, green beans, garlic, seaweed

Miscellaneous: molasses

Eat whole grains rather than refined ones, as the refining of grains can reduce selenium content from 50 to 70%. In addition, soils vary dramatically in their selenium content, and a plant's ability to absorb this mineral from the soil can be inhibited by sulfur in fertilizer and acid rain.

Zinc

BENEFITS

- Helps maintain skin, hair, and nails

- Essential for bone health

- As an antioxidant, frees vitamin A to prevent night blindness, which can become more common with age

- Nourishes sexuality

- Supports the functioning of every body system due to its role in working with enzymes to catalyze chemical reactions

BEST FOOD SOURCES OF ZINC

Nuts: Brazil nuts, cashews, pecans, peanuts

Seeds: pumpkin, sesame, sunflower

Seafood: oysters, crab, lobster, herring

Meat: liver, beef

Poultry: turkey

Vegetables: corn, mushrooms, seaweed

Beans: chickpeas, white, soy, black-eyed peas

Grains: brown rice, whole wheat

Miscellaneous: eggs

Taking Supplements

As you pass through menopause and your body attempts to meet the challenge of your changing body chemistry, you may require higher levels of certain nutrients. If you were in the habit of eating very nutritious foods, your diet may have delivered your daily requirement. But with menopause, you may need higher doses of certain vitamins, minerals, and phytonutrients than can be supplied by the quantity of food you eat. In this case, supplements are the answer.

Nutrient Ratios

Supplemental vitamins and minerals should be present in proportion with one another, just as they are in food. For instance, figs supply both calcium and magnesium, two minerals that counterbalance each other within the body. If you decide to take one of these as a supplement, you need to make sure you also have sufficient amounts of the other. Theories vary about the best ratio, but usually calcium and magnesium are supplemented in a 2:1 ratio, for instance, 1000 milligrams of calcium, and 500 milligrams of magnesium.

Eating a varied diet can supply you with a fairly balanced mix of nutrients. However, despite your best intentions, you may not always eat as you should. In this case, take a multivitamin/mineral supplement. These formulated supplements provide nutrients in carefully determined ratios.

General Recommendations of Vitamins and Minerals for Menopause

The following list of recommended vitamins and minerals gives the minimum dosage that may be helpful as well as the maximum dosage usually recommended, although some have a higher limit for certain individuals. These amounts are many times greater than the recommended daily allowances (RDAs) because these nutrients are being used in a therapeutic way to prevent and treat symptoms.

You can find many menopausal vitamin and mineral supplements sold in vitamin shops and natural food stores. The dosages of specific nutrients in these supplements will likely fall into the ranges given here. Use this chart to check the ingredient list on the bottle for effective and safe amounts.

If you feel you need to take a more individualized mix of nutrients than standard formulas provide, take care not to exceed the maximum doses listed. Even better, consult with your physician or a nutritionist. Trained professionals can order blood tests and hair analyses to assess the levels of certain nutrients within your body. Based on test results and taking your menopause symptoms into consideration, they should be able to give you an informed recommendation of what you need.

To enjoy the benefits of taking supplements, you have to first swallow them! You may take supplements for a while and feel so good that you stop. Once you have a protocol that seems to be working for you, stick with it.

Vitamins and Minerals	Dosages for Menopause
Vitamin A (retinol)	5000–10,000 IU
Vitamin A (from beta-carotene)	10,000–75,000 IU
Thiamin (vitamin B_1)	10–90 mg
Riboflavin (vitamin B_2)	10–90 mg
Niacin (vitamin B_3)	10–90 mg
Pyridoxine (vitamin B_6)	25–200 mg
Biotin	100–300 mcg
Pantothenic acid (vitamin B_5)	25–100 mg
Folic acid	400–1000 mcg
Cobalamin (vitamin B_{12})	400–1000 mcg
Choline	150–500 mg
Inositol	150–500 mg
Vitamin C	1000–4000 mg
Vitamin D	100–400 IU
Vitamin E (tocopherol)	400–1600 IU
Vitamin K	60–900 mcg
Boron	3–5 mg
Calcium	250–1200 mg
Chromium	200–400 mcg
Copper	1–2 mg
Iodine	50–200 mcg
Iron	15–20 mg
Magnesium	250–750 mg
Manganese	10–15 mg
Molybdenum	10–25 mcg
Potassium	100–500 mg
Selenium	100–250 mg
Silica	200–1000 mcg
Vanadium	50–100 mcg
Zinc	15–30 mg

Choosing the Best Form of Key Nutrients

If you shop for supplements, you'll find that vitamin C comes in capsules but is also available as a powder. Natural vitamin E is on the market, but stores also sell synthetic vitamin E. Minerals are not sold in their pure form. Rather, bottles list calcium as calcium carbonate or calcium citrate. This section explains which forms of these nutrients are the most beneficial.

Vitamin C

Vitamin C is an acid—ascorbic acid—and in high doses it can cause gastric discomfort. An alternative that is less acidic is sold in powder form under the trade name Ester-C ascorbate, which is more easily absorbed than regular vitamin C and is better utilized by body tissues. Another bonus of Ester-C ascorbate is that it does not erode tooth enamel. Plain ascorbic acid can cause severe damage to teeth, especially if you take chewable vitamin C, which comes in direct contact with your teeth. For insurance, whenever you take any form of vitamin C, be sure to rinse your mouth afterward with filtered water.

Vitamin C remains in your system for only about 4 hours before it is excreted in the urine. For this reason, take vitamin C in divided doses throughout the day. The first sign of overdosing is diarrhea.

Vitamin E

Natural vitamin E is made from vegetable oils and consists of one particular type of molecule, called d-alpha tocopherol. Some natural vitamin E supplements also contain mixed tocopherols. These are beta, gamma, and delta tocopherols, which have less vitamin E activity in the body but are also beneficial.

Synthetic vitamin E is made from petroleum or turpentine and is a mixture of eight molecular configurations, seven of which are man-made and do not occur in nature. Synthetic vitamin E is referred to as dl-alpha tocopherol.

Natural vitamin E appears to be more beneficial than synthetic vitamin E in that it is better absorbed into organs and tissues. In addition, some researchers question whether synthetic vitamin E actually ties up receptor sites, preventing any natural vitamin E present from acting. To be sure your vitamin E is 100% natural, look for the following on the label: independently assayed to guarantee 100% potency, 100% natural source.

As vitamin E is an oil-soluble vitamin, there is the possibility of overdosing and toxicity. Signs of toxicity include nausea, diarrhea, intestinal gas, headache, heart palpitations, and fainting. Dosages recommended for menopause are many times greater than the RDA. However, even in these greater quantities, signs of toxicity are rare.

To gauge how much vitamin E you can tolerate while taking a sufficient amount to decrease menopausal symptoms, increase your intake slowly. Begin with 400 international units a day and continue this for 2 weeks, then add another 400 international units every 2 weeks, until you notice symptoms such as hot flashes subsiding. Stop increasing the dosage when it reaches 1600 international units a day. If you decide to cut back, reduce your intake by 400 international units in 2-week intervals.

Calcium

Calcium carbonate provides the most concentrated form of calcium. It is adequately absorbed if taken with meals. Look for kinds that are factory made, rather than natural calcium carbonate in the form of bone meal, oyster shell, or dolomite, which may contain lead.

Other forms of calcium supplements include calcium phosphate, calcium lactate, calcium gluconate, calcium maleate, and, most importantly, calcium citrate. This form of calcium is much better absorbed than other forms and is widely available. However, one drawback of calcium citrate is that it can increase the absorption of aluminum, a mineral that may lead to kidney disease and is linked to Alzheimer's disease. If you take calcium in this form, make sure the deodorant you are using does not contain aluminum. In addition, avoid eating food cooked in aluminum pots and pans. Note that some restaurants such as diners use this cheaper type of cookware.

If you want to check on how easily your calcium supplement dissolves, indicating how easily it may be absorbed, place a calcium tablet in 6 ounces of white vinegar or apple cider vinegar. Set this aside for 30 minutes, stirring occasionally. A top-quality calcium tablet should dissolve within this period.

For maximum absorption, take calcium in divided doses, two to three times a day. With each dose, also take some vitamin C, which increases absorption of this important mineral. Some people find that calcium makes them feel relaxed and even drowsy, so you may want to take it before bedtime.

Special Nutrients

Besides the familiar vitamins and minerals just described, nature provides other key nutrients to assist your passage through menopause. These nutrients include bioflavonoids, compounds similar to vitamins; phytoestrogens, substances that behave like hormones within the body; and essential fatty acids, a group of fats that promote good health.

Many common foods contain these nutrients, but a diet of fast foods only provides a meager amount. To ensure an adequate intake, you need to turn to the simple fare of whole foods described in Chapter 5. For now, let's take a look at these nutrients, what they consist of, and how they behave within your body tissues.

oids

...iavonoids, originally called P vitamins, are not actually vitamins. They are a group of water-soluble compounds that include such substances as citrin, hesperidin, quercetin, rutin, flavones, and flavonols. Some combination of these is often included in vitamin supplements for women.

In foods, bioflavonoids are accompanied by vitamin C, a combination that allows for better absorption of the bioflavonoids. Citrus is an especially rich source of these vitamins, with lemons containing the entire complex. The central fluffy white stem within citrus fruits contains the highest concentration of bioflavonoids.

The chemical formula of certain bioflavonoids resembles that of estradiol, the primary form of estrogen. These bioflavonoids display chemical activity similar to this hormone.

BENEFITS

Bioflavonoids help control hot flashes. They are also used to lessen the psychological symptoms of menopause, including anxiety, irritability, and mood swings. Bioflavonoids strengthen capillary walls, thereby curbing heavy menstrual bleeding that can occur during perimenopause. This action also helps reduce the likelihood of varicose veins, spider veins, hemorrhages, and black-and-blue marks. Rutin is particularly effective in preventing varicose veins. Bioflavonoids help slow the aging process in other ways too. They work in conjunction with vitamin C to prevent ruptures in connective tissue, keeping skin firm and healthy. And the bioflavonoid quercetin helps prevent cataracts.

GOOD FOOD SOURCES OF BIOFLAVONOIDS

Fruit: black currants; grapes; plums; cherries; apricots; blackberries; papaya; cantaloupe; the pith, membranes, and central white core of citrus including oranges, lemons, limes, and grapefruit

Vegetables: green peppers, tomatoes, broccoli

Whole grains: buckwheat

Miscellaneous: rose hips

COOKING TIPS

- Bioflavonoids are very stable compounds, minimally affected by heat, air, and light. They are present even in canned fruits and vegetables.

Phytoestrogens: Hormones from the Plant Kingdom

Many common foods contain compounds that have the capability of behaving like hormones within the human body. These have been given the popular name of *phytoestrogens*. Such compounds first drew the attention of scientists in the 1940s when it was observed that sheep in many parts of Australia were becoming infertile. The ewes stopped ovulating. The problem was eventually traced to the red clover on which the sheep were grazing. Red clover, as explained in Chapter 6, contains especially high amounts of estrogenic isoflavones. The animals were taking in about 1 gram a day, a very large amount. Such extremely high doses can stop ovulation. Birth-control pills function the same way.

By the 1970s, attention turned to the effects of estrogens in the human diet. Scientists began measuring the phytohormone content of dozens of vegetables, fruits, grains, seeds, and flavorings routinely used in cooking that show some degree of estrogenic activity. These days the research focus is on the effect of all these phytoestrogen-rich foods on symptoms of menopause. In addition, their potential ability to lower the risk of heart disease and breast cancer is being addressed.

Why Phytoestrogens Are Important for Female Health

Phytoestrogens function as modulators and have a balancing effect on hormone levels. They play a dual role, mimicking the functions of estrogen when supply is low and dampening it when too much is available. Phytoestrogens bind to estrogen receptor sites, such as those found in breast tissue. This blocks the body's own more potent form of estrogen from attaching, and because of the lower potency of phytoestrogens, this substitution in effect reduces estrogenic activity. But when the body is producing only a small amount of estrogen, plant estrogens make a contribution to this supply.

However, as Bruce Milliman, N.D., associate professor adjunct faculty at Bastyr University in Seattle, states, "The impact of phytoestrogens on the system goes way beyond their activity at binding sites. They can also mimic estrogen as well as impeding the breakdown of estrogen." And, he continues, "In addition, the functions of phytoestrogens may also depend on the ratio of various types of estrogens within a woman's body. And diet can be an important part of the equation. So the questions and answers are very complicated."

Subtle Potency But Powerful Effects

Although estrogenic substances in foods have been shown to affect hormone status, phytoestrogens have potencies that are far, far weaker when compared with the effectiveness of estradiol, the primary form of estrogen made by the ovaries. Phytoestrogens have only 1/400 to 1/100,000 the potency of estradiol.

However, certain ways of eating can provide a significant amount of phytoestrogenic ingredients, which can make a difference. In a landmark study, women living in rural Japan who ate a diet high in estrogenic soy foods were found to have levels of phytoestrogens in their urine in quantities 100 to 1000 times greater than that of women in the United States. Japanese women have a much lower incidence of hot flashes: fewer than 20% of them compared with 80% of North American women experience this symptom. In fact, the Japanese language doesn't even include a word for "hot flash." Various studies have also shown that women who eat a vegetarian diet may have phytoestrogen levels 100 times greater than women eating a typical North American diet.

COMMON FOODS THAT CONTAIN COMPOUNDS
WITH ESTROGENIC ACTIVITY

Many foods supply phytoestrogens:

- *Grains.*   A variety of grains show estrogenic activity, but you need to eat these in their unrefined, whole form: whole wheat, brown rice, oats, barley, rye, cornmeal.

- *Vegetables.*   Some of the most common produce has estrogenic activity. This list also makes a good salad: cucumbers, radishes, carrots, parsley, onions, green beans, cabbage, potatoes, sugar beets, peas.

- *Fruit.*   Pomegranates, an ancient symbol of fertility, are an estrogenic fruit; so are cherries, rhubarb, apples, and citrus fruits.

- *Seeds.*   In Ethiopia, a country in which menopause is not nearly as troublesome for women as in the West, estrogenic flaxseeds are included in many forms and in many dishes throughout the year. Oils from seeds, as well as nuts, contain phytohormones, if the oils remain natural and unrefined. Studies show that flaxseed functions as a menstrual regulator. Flax helps to ensure that a woman ovulates each month and that progesterone and estrogen production remain in balance. This in turn can lower the risk of certain conditions that are associated with unopposed estrogen, such as PMS, the growth of fibroids, and breast cancer. Sesame seeds are also a good source of phytoestrogens.

- *Cooking herbs and seasonings.* These various estrogenic flavorings have long been used by herbalists to support female health: licorice, garlic, fennel, sage, and anise.

- *Beverages.* Many women are switching from coffee and regular black tea to the Asian staple, green tea, which contains phytoestrogens.

- *Legumes.* Beans, peas, and lentils contain especially high levels of estrogenic compounds. If you eat navy beans, chickpeas, black-eyed peas, or lentils, you will be taking in estrogenic isoflavones. Soybeans in particular contain an especially potent form of isoflavones, specifically genistein and daidzein.

THE YAM AND SWEET POTATO MIXUP

The Mexican wild yam, which is inedible, is exceptionally high in phytohormones. Compounds derived from this type of yam were used to make the first birth-control pills. Today, progesterone supplements are made from this plant, which has received much attention with all the interest in natural treatments for menopause. In ethnic markets, you may find a type of yam, thin skinned and often weighing several pounds, a staple of African and Caribbean cooking, but this yam does not contain estrogenic compounds. Then there are sweet potatoes, the size of the common baking potato. They have a rough skin and either orange or pale yellow flesh. Sweet potatoes are available in most supermarkets and are often mislabeled "yams," and these too have no effect on hormones.

Essential Fatty Acids

Essential fatty acids are special fats that the body requires for normal functioning. Although plants can manufacture essential fatty acids, we can't—we must get our supply from what we eat. There are two families of EFAs: omega-6 and omega-3. You'll also hear these referred to as linoleic acid and linolenic acid, respectively. Omega-6 EFAs are plentiful in most seeds and nuts, and the cooking oils made from these; omega-3 EFAs are plentiful in walnuts, flaxseeds, flaxseed oil, and fatty fish such as salmon and tuna.

Getting enough EFAs is an intrinsic part of caring for yourself before and during menopause, because the EFAs are components of many tissues and organs that are stressed or undergoing changes at this time. They play a role in the functioning of the adrenals, the sex glands, brain cells, and skin tissue, and also help maintain the orderly sequence of the heartbeat. EFAs have been shown to help prevent heart disease and breast cancer.

It's thought that a healthful ratio of omega-6 to omega-3 is approximately 2:1. The North American diet, high in plant seed oils, radically tips this balance so that the estimated ratio is 20:1. While suffering the effects of too much omega-6, we're missing the health-giving properties of omega-3. (For more about EFAs, see Chapter 5.)

As you increase your intake of essential fatty acids, you must also increase your intake of antioxidants, that is, vitamin C, beta-carotene, vitamin E, and selenium. EFAs are unstable molecules that easily break down in the presence of oxygen, light, and heat and generate free radicals. Free radicals attack cell structures and are thought to be the primary reason for aging. Antioxidants stop these molecules from doing damage.

Now that you've been introduced to the range of nutrients that can help support your health at menopause, let's take a look at the eating style that can help guarantee an easy menopause. The following chapter covers the basic food groups and gives you a helping hand in the kitchen with suggestions for healthy everyday meals.

NUTRIENTS FOR THE SYMPTOMS OF MENOPAUSE

Hot flashes: niacin, pantothenic acid, vitamin C, vitamin E, chromium, magnesium, potassium, selenium, bioflavonoids, phytoestrogens, essential fatty acids

Fatigue: niacin, pantothenic acid, vitamin B_{12}, folic acid, vitamin C, vitamin E, calcium, iodine, iron, magnesium, manganese, potassium

Mood swings: riboflavin, vitamin B_5, chromium, bioflavonoids, phytoestrogens

Anxiety and irritability: thiamin, riboflavin, pantothenic acid, folic acid, vitamin C, vitamin D, vitamin E, calcium, copper, magnesium, manganese, phosphorus, potassium, bioflavonoids, essential fatty acids

Depression: vitamin B_6, magnesium

Poor memory: thiamin, niacin, pantothenic acid, vitamin B_{12}, folic acid, iodine, essential fatty acids

Vaginal thinning and loss of elasticity: vitamin A, riboflavin, niacin, vitamin B_6, vitamin C, vitamin E, copper, selenium, essential fatty acids

Vaginal lubrication: niacin, vitamin C, vitamin E, selenium

Libido: zinc

Fluid retention: vitamin B_6

Irregular cycles: phytoestrogens

Heavy menstrual flow: bioflavonoids, vitamin C

CHAPTER FIVE

Step 2: Diet and Menopause— The Way to Eat

Because nutrient-rich foods provide a foundation for good health, eating nourishing foods makes up the second step of the Healthy Menopause Program. However, as basic as eating well is to good health, diet is not usually emphasized in medical protocols. If you consult a conventional physician about lessening symptoms of menopause, you are most likely to be offered hormone replacement therapy (HRT) as a first line of defense.

One important advantage of using food as a way of preventing menopause symptoms is that food is not likely to cause side effects. The same cannot be said of hormone replacement therapy (see Chapter 9). And even if you take supplemental hormones, you still have to eat. Find out all you can about foods for menopause and those that should be avoided, starting with the following information.

The Standard Diet and Menopause

Many of the most commonly eaten foods can undermine your health and make your passage through menopause more difficult. The great majority of meals contain some form of refined wheat and refined white sugar. In fact, the average American consumes approximately 155 pounds of sugar each year. Vegetables are scarce and meats and fried foods are ample. To make matters worse, the meal is often washed down with a cola and topped off with caffeinated coffee to rev up the system after this energy-depleting repast.

Nutritionist Vesanto Melina, R.D., sees the effects of such a diet in her practice. As she reports:

> The women I consult with who have been eating an average American diet have a fair amount of trouble with menopause. But it's another story with women who are more the health food types. They've been exercising, and they aren't overly fat, and because of what they have been eating, their bodies are prepared and are not toxic. When it comes to menopause, these women are just cruising through.

Sugar

When you eat sugars, including refined white sugar, maple syrup, and honey, your body metabolizes these to glucose, a simple sugar that circulates in the blood. Glucose is a source of energy and the only fuel that the brain can use. For normal functioning, you need a fairly steady level of blood glucose. In susceptible individuals, the ability to manage glucose levels can diminish with age and it may be that problems attributed to menopause at midlife also involve glucose metabolism. Low blood sugar stresses the system and can trigger a variety of symptoms, including anxiety, fatigue, poor memory, and even hot flashes. As a normal blood glucose level is restored, the effects are just as dramatic, with evidence of increased energy and mental clarity.

Steadying Blood Glucose

You can do much to steady your blood sugar levels by following these simple guidelines:

- Be sure to eat three meals a day at regular intervals, beginning with breakfast.

- Have a snack between meals if you feel your blood sugar dropping.

- Be sure to include carbohydrates, proteins, and fats in your diet. Each of these food groups provides energy at a different rate. By eating all three at the same time, you help ensure that you will have an even supply of blood sugar over about a 3-hour period. Carbohydrates break down in about 1½ hours, protein after 2 to 2½ hours, and fats after 3 hours.

Fiber

Estrogens produced by the body eventually leave the body via the intestinal tract. As they pass through the large intestine, some may combine with other compounds, and, in this form, eventually be reabsorbed back into the system. However, fiber intake appears to help control the level of estrogens in the blood by promoting its excretion. A diet high in fiber may help reduce symptoms of menopause associated with high levels of estrogen, such as anxiety, as well as the risk of breast cancer, which is also associated with this type of hormone imbalance.

Colas

Colas contain sugar, caffeine, and phosphoric acid, a cocktail of substances that can undermine female health. Besides the effects of sugar already described, the caffeine in cola stresses the adrenal glands, which are an important source of sex hormones after menopause. Overworked adrenal glands appear to be involved in hormonal imbalances that can bring on menopausal symptoms. (Caffeinated coffee and teas have the same effect.) And phosphoric acid can increase levels of phosphorus in the bloodstream, causing calcium to be pulled from the skeletal system, thereby setting the stage for osteoporosis to develop.

Improving Your Diet

If you've been skipping breakfast and having fast-food lunches, with a sudden improvement in diet you may feel better in just days. Hot flashes brought on by having a Danish pastry and a strong cup of caffeinated coffee abate as soon as the offending foods are cut from the diet. However, fully restoring your hormonal health as well as vitality and general well-being may take 2 to 3 months or even longer. You need to increase your body stores of vitamins, minerals, and other nutrients.

Once you build up your nutrient reserves and begin to feel better, you may be tempted to return to your old ways. You may have a grace period during which it's easy to think that it doesn't matter what you eat and that you are through the worst of menopause anyway. But continue your previous habits for a week or two and menopausal symptoms are likely to recur— it's a good way to test how bad some foods can make you feel!

Whole Foods

Eating for menopause can be a pleasure. The freshest, most natural, and beautifully colored ingredients are just what you need. Golden squash, ruby-red berries, the season's best peaches and figs, glistening fresh fish, raw nuts and seeds, and frilly herbs are on the menu! These foods and others like them are rich sources of the many nutrients important for menopause that were presented in Chapter 4. These ingredients all have something in common. They are whole foods—foods with all their parts, such as beets plus their tops, potatoes with their skins. These foods are also unrefined, unprocessed, and free of added chemicals, artificial flavors, and coloring agents.

You can find whole foods at your regular supermarket, in natural food stores, and at farmers' markets. The price of fresh food can sometimes seem expensive, especially if it is organic, but such foods cost less, pound for pound, than foods that have been refined, altered, and elaborately packaged and advertised. For some food products, nearly 75% of each dollar you spend may go to the manufacturer's costs, not the food itself.

Traditional Foods versus the Modern Diet

Women in many parts of the world, from the Mediterranean coast and Africa, to India and Japan, describe a menopause that is relatively free of symptoms compared to the difficulties women in North America experience. One reason these various populations fare better is that traditional and whole foods still make up a significant part of their diet. Meals are made from staples such as lentils, whole grains, fresh nuts and seeds, and seasonal fruits and vegetables. Fish is eaten far more frequently than in North America, and red meat and poultry are consumed in smaller portions. Particularly in less developed countries and in more rural areas, meals are likely to be made up of simple fare. People cook with ingredients that are grown locally and are often less processed. Consequently, such foods are likely to contain higher levels of nutrients and fewer harmful chemicals.

Plant Foods to the Rescue

Eating a vegetarian or mostly vegetarian diet is associated with fewer menopausal symptoms. As women's health specialist, Susan M. Lark, M.D., recommends, "For optimal health, women need to eat a plant foods–based diet, emphasizing whole grains, legumes including beans and peas, raw seeds and nuts, and lots of fruits and vegetables. And if a woman wants to eat animals foods, fish is a better choice than red meat or poultry." Dr. Lark continues, "There is evidence that women who follow this type of program can reduce and prevent menopause symptoms. These foods are great sources of phytoestrogens, minerals such as calcium and magnesium, and essential fatty acids, all important for a woman's health."

A survey conducted for *Prevention* magazine in 1993 supports these recommendations. The research, headed by Fredi Kronenberg, Ph.D., director of menopause research at the Center for Women's Health at Columbia-Presbyterian Medical Center, New York City, assessed the relationship of menopausal symptoms to diet and found that women who were vegetarians or who ate mostly vegetarian foods reported significantly fewer symptoms than women who only occasionally if ever had vegetarian meals. In addition, soy foods were associated with fewer symptoms. One explanation for these apparent benefits may be that women who are vegetarians and/or eat soy live a healthier lifestyle in general. Another explanation is that such a diet supplies a greater amount of phytoestrogens, which help even out hormones that can bring on symptoms when out of balance. (See Chapter 4 for more on phytoestrogens.)

According to a study published in the *British Medical Journal* in 1990, researchers in Melbourne, Australia, found that supplementing women's diets with estrogenic foods resulted in signs of an estrogen response. (For experimental purposes, this is measured by microscopic examination of vaginal cells.

The vaginal wall thickens as the amount of estrogen in the system increases.) In the study, the estrogenic foods made up about 10% of the women's diet. However, as the study points out, in some parts of the world, estrogenic plants provide 50% of calories women consume each day. A diet so abundant in phytoestrogens may play a significant role in diminishing menopausal symptoms.

Organic Foods

Organic food is grown without pesticides, herbicides, or chemical fertilizers on land that has been free of chemicals for at least 3 preceding years. Fertilizers and mulches must consist only of animal and vegetable matter. "Certified" organic is a guarantee that an independent organization has inspected some combination of the produce, the soil, and the grower's methods, and has made sure that they meet the established standard.

Although plant food can be only as nutrient rich as the soil in which it was grown, there is some evidence that organic foods may contain higher levels of vitamins and minerals. An often cited study is "Organic Foods vs. Supermarket Foods: Element Levels," published in 1993 in the *Journal of Applied Nutrition*. Organic pears, apples, potatoes, and wheat sampled over a 2-year period contained an average of 90% more nutrients than similar commercial nonorganic foods. This nutrient bonus, often available in organic foods, is just what women need as they approach menopause.

Insecticides such as endosulfan and methoxychlor that are widely used on crops are classed as estrogen-like compounds. Whereas the body quickly breaks down phytoestrogens naturally present in plant foods, synthetic estrogens tend to build up in the blood and fatty tissue over time. The effect of these chemicals may be sufficient to upset a woman's hormone balance and help trigger menopausal symptoms. There may also be a link between synthetic estrogens and breast cancer, a further reason to shop for organic foods.

Although some dangerous pesticides have been banned in North America, these same pesticides continue to be sold to farmers in other countries, especially Central and South America. Crops treated with these return to North America and are sold in grocery stores. Such produce makes up about 10% of total intake of fruits and vegetables, a figure that may be even higher in northern regions during winter months when local crops are not available.

Some toxins in the environment, although not estrogenic, are capable of interfering with the reproductive system. Dioxin, which is an unintentional by-product of many industrial processes involving chlorine, is a known human carcinogen and can cause severe reproductive problems. Dioxin is in commonly eaten foods such as beef, milk and other dairy products, chicken, and pork, and to a lesser extent fish and eggs. It is fat-soluble and moves up the food chain.

Fortunately more stores are making organic foods available. If the produce buyer or butcher in your neighborhood market has not yet begun offering this choice, take the initiative and explain that you want more female-friendly foods!

The Best Foods for Menopause

Within every category of food, from grains to beverages, certain foods are especially abundant in nutrients for menopause. Take a look at the following items and begin to include the recommended foods in your shopping list.

Whole Grains

Whole grains are a source of vitamin E, one of the most important nutrients for discouraging hot flashes. They supply B vitamins that nourish the nervous system and help steady emotions. In addition, because whole grains are digested more slowly than refined grains, these foods are less likely to trigger abrupt changes in blood sugar and thus trigger symptoms.

When grain is refined, the wheat germ is removed along with the healthy oils, B vitamins, and vitamin E. When this refined grain is used to make bread, manufacturers enrich the grain, but only some of the original nutrients are returned. Refined wheat, as compared with whole wheat, contains less vitamin E, magnesium, calcium, copper, iron, phosphorus, potassium, selenium, and zinc, and even lower amounts of some of the B vitamins with which it is enriched. Refining also removes fiber, which helps balance hormones.

GRAIN PRESCRIPTION

Be sure to eat a variety of grains such as oats and millet, and grains such as quinoa, a staple of early civilizations in South America. And enjoy buckwheat, which is not really a grain but the seed of an herb. Buckwheat supplies estrogenic bioflavonoids. In eastern European countries and in Russia, buckwheat is eaten as kasha, and Japanese cook with soba noodles that are made of buckwheat. Choose from among the following: oats, barley, rye, brown rice, whole-wheat couscous, bulgur wheat, millet, cornmeal, quinoa, amaranthe, kamut.

SHOPPING FOR WHOLE GRAINS

Look for labels that specifically state "whole grain," which means that the flour was not refined. Whole wheat is not whole grain. Whole-wheat bread usually has as its first ingredient some form of refined wheat flour. These days, you can find whole-grain bagels, English muffins, and croissants. In natural food stores, you can also find whole-grain hot breakfast cereal, such as cream of whole wheat, cream of brown rice, and cream of buckwheat. Some natural food stores even carry whole-grain croutons and ready-made bread crumbs.

Legumes

Legumes, that is, beans, lentils, and peas, are a mineral-rich, low-fat source of protein, which is just what you want in your diet as you approach midlife. Your body needs the minerals to help maintain strong bones and manage stress, and reducing your fat intake can help you curb the weight gain that can occur as your sex hormone production changes. Beans are also high in water-soluble fiber, which can help lower cholesterol.

LEGUME PRESCRIPTION

Beans are eaten less frequently than years ago. To increase your intake, include them in soups and salads. Soybeans are particularly high in phytoestrogens. Choose from among the following: navy beans, pinto beans, black beans, lima beans, lentils, black-eyed peas, chickpeas, soybeans.

Vegetables and Fruit

One of the Dietary Guidelines for Americans is to eat at least five servings a day of fruits and vegetables. As Hugh Riordan, M.D., says, "It's generally thought that if you were to eat the recommended minimum of five servings a day, you might indeed have good levels of vitamins and minerals in your body. But the current estimate is that less than 9% of the population eats this much. This means that probably a lot of women begin menopause missing important nutrients that they need." To increase your intake, snack on fruit at work. In restaurants, order a salad that includes a variety of vegetables. At home, cook vegetable soups.

When you shop for produce, invest in the best quality you can find. Whenever possible, buy fresh local fruits and vegetables. Local produce can be more nutritious and is less likely to be treated with preservatives used to keep produce fresh while being transported long distances to market. It's also likely to be higher in nutrients, which the rigors of shipping can destroy.

And if you buy local produce at a farmers' market, you have the opportunity to talk directly to the grower and check whether the produce was sprayed with pesticides.

VEGETABLE PRESCRIPTION

Some vegetables are particularly high in nutrients that support health during and postmenopause. However, the best advice is to eat a variety of vegetables, which can supply you with a range of nutrients. Choose from among the following: red onions, asparagus, artichokes, winter squash, broccoli, green beans, celery, sweet red peppers, garlic, parsley, tomatoes, kale.

ARE YOU REALLY EATING A VARIETY OF VEGETABLES?

Many women sincerely think they eat quite a variety of vegetables, but actually they do not. Check your own eating habits against this table that starts in the left-hand column with the most commonly eaten vegetables. Then take a look at the other two columns of vegetables that are eaten less frequently. How many vegetables do you usually eat from the middle and right-hand lists?

Commonly Eaten	*Eaten Less Frequently*	*Eaten Rarely*
potatoes	broccoli	winter squash
corn	green beans	asparagus
peas	mushrooms	broccoli rabe
tomatoes	beets	brussels sprouts
carrots	spinach	kale
celery	cauliflower	collards
zucchini	peppers	turnip greens
iceberg lettuce	cabbage	Chinese cabbage
	sweet potatoes	bok choy
	watercress	artichokes
	romaine	arugula

Fruit Prescription

Fruit is an excellent source of fiber, minerals, and special nutrients for menopause such as bioflavonoids. The following fruits are especially rich sources: berries, citrus, apples, melons, currants, avocado, mango, papaya, plantain.

Are You Really Eating a Variety of Fruit?

Eating a variety of fruit is also essential for lasting health. Check your intake using this table.

Commonly Eaten	*Eaten Less Frequently*	*Eaten Rarely*
apples	grapes	apricots
bananas	strawberries	blackberries
oranges	cantaloupe	raspberries
lemons	prunes	limes
pears	peaches	kiwi
watermelon	raisins	tangerines
	pineapple	currants
	grapefruit	plantain
	blueberries	mango
	avocado	papaya
		plums
		cherimoya
		dates

THE DIRTY DOZEN

The Environmental Working Group (EWG), a nonprofit environmental research organization, assembled a list of 12 fruits and vegetables that have been found to contain the highest levels of pesticides. The EWG estimates that by avoiding these foods or by choosing organically grown varieties you can cut your health risk from pesticides by about 50%. Take a look at the following list, which also gives you alternatives that supply some of the same nutrients.

1. Strawberries. *Alternatives:* blackberries, raspberries, blueberries, citrus fruit such as oranges and grapefruit, watermelon, U.S.-grown cantaloupe and kiwi

2. Bell peppers. *Alternatives:* romaine lettuce, broccoli, peas, tomatoes, carrots, broccoli, asparagus, brussels sprouts

3. Spinach. *Alternatives:* asparagus, brussels sprouts, romaine lettuce, broccoli

4. U.S.-grown cherries. *Alternatives:* blueberries, blackberries, oranges, grapefruit, kiwi, U.S.-grown cantaloupe

5. Peaches. *Alternatives:* nectarines, red or pink grapefruit, oranges, tangerines, watermelon, U.S.–grown cantaloupe

6. Mexican-grown cantaloupe. *Alternatives:* U.S.-grown cantaloupe, watermelon

7. Celery. *Alternatives:* radishes, carrots, broccoli, romaine lettuce

8. Apples. *Alternatives:* citrus including oranges, grapefruit, and tangerines, nectarines, bananas, pears, kiwi, watermelon, U.S.-grown cantaloupe

9. Apricots. *Alternatives:* red or pink grapefruit, oranges, tangerines, nectarines, U.S.-grown cantaloupe, watermelon

10. Green beans. *Alternatives:* broccoli, peas, cauliflower, potatoes, asparagus, brussels sprouts

11. Grapes from Chile. *Alternatives:* U.S.-grown grapes available in season from May to December

12. Cucumbers. *Alternatives:* carrots, broccoli, radishes, romaine lettuce

Meat and Poultry

Although many women in menopause feel best eating a vegetarian or mostly vegetarian diet, animal protein, including meat and poultry, can have a place in a menopause diet. These foods supply protein, which your body requires daily, since protein is not stored. According to the U.S. Department of Agriculture's Food Guide Pyramid, you need two to three servings a day of protein food from a variety of sources: meat, poultry, fish, dry beans, eggs, and nuts. (Not included in the protein section of the pyramid are vegetables and grains, which are also good sources of protein.)

Recommended portion sizes for meat are smaller than you might think: only 4 ounces. Four ounces of hamburger is the size of a pack of cards—hardly the American standard for a serving of steak! However, such modest portions are just what is needed if you top a salad with strips of grilled chicken breast or add chunks of beef to a bean and vegetable soup—both excellent menu choices for menopause.

Choosing lean cuts of meat is also important to help manage weight and limit the intake of saturated fats that meat contains. Lean and round cuts of meat, such as pork loin and white-meat chicken rather than dark meat, have less fat. Visible fat should be trimmed from meat and poultry.

Meat and poultry are good sources of B vitamins and many minerals needed for good health. In particular, meat is an excellent source of vitamin B_{12}, an energy nutrient essential for normal functioning of the nervous system; and iron, an oxygen-carrying component of blood. Heavy menstrual flow can cause iron to become depleted, causing fatigue.

You may also want to schedule *when* you eat meat according to your menstrual cycle. Red meat, and to a lesser degree pork and poultry, contain arachidonic acid, a substance that can lead to menstrual cramps, which occur in some women as they develop erratic periods during perimenopause. If you suffer from menstrual cramps, stay away from meat as well as dairy foods for at least a few days preceding and during your menstrual cycle.

CHOOSE "CLEAN" MEATS

Go out of your way to buy meat raised without added hormones. These hormones can alter the balance of your own hormones and may contribute to menopausal symptoms. Look for meats that are labeled "residue-free."

Fish and Shellfish

Seafood, including fish and shellfish, is an excellent source of minerals. Seafood supplies iodine, magnesium, manganese, copper, phosphorus, and notably selenium, a trace mineral that is lacking in the standard North American diet. Selenium boosts the benefits of vitamin E, a nutrient vital for menopausal health. Seafood is also a source of the fat-soluble vitamins A, D, and E.

In addition, seafood is an excellent source of omega-3 fatty acids—quality fats that play a vital role in female health postmenopause. Omega-3 helps maintain vaginal health, skin quality, and good memory. Richer-tasting, oilier fish contain the highest amounts, for example, salmon, tuna, mackerel, herring, and anchovies. Caviar is also a superb source!

Make an effort to eat fish two or three times a week to benefit from this exceptionally healthy source of nutrients. However, eating seafood more frequently than this can have its drawbacks. Because of polluted waters, seafood can contain heavy metals and other toxins. Limit your exposure by eating a variety of seafood, and eat smaller fish that are lower on the food chain and are less likely to concentrate toxins, and eat offshore fish such as sole, cod, and tuna.

Fats and Oils

Fat is feared because eating too much can put on pounds, especially postmenopause when most women tend to gain weight. Indeed, the average North American consumes too many calories from fat, about 40% of calories rather than the 30% recommended by the American Heart Association. However, quality fats are actually an essential part of a healthy diet. Fat helps the body stay warm. Fat insulates the nerves and provides cushioning to protect organs. And fat is the raw material from which hormones are made.

Health does not depend on the quantity of fat consumed but the quality. The healthiest fats and oils on the market are:

Extra-virgin olive oil

Unrefined safflower oil

Unrefined sesame oil

Flaxseed oil

Organic, unsalted butter

Monounsaturated fats, such as olive oil, are associated with lower rates of heart disease, while saturated fats, found in butter and coconut oil, can clog arteries. When eaten in excess, polyunsaturated fats, such as canola, safflower, and grapeseed oil, fall somewhere in between, lowering low-density lipoprotein (LDL), the bad cholesterol, but also high-density lipoprotein (HDL), the good cholesterol. Some of each of these kinds of fat has a place in a healthy diet, with an emphasis on the monounsaturates and polyunsaturates.

REACH FOR OILS THAT ARE UNREFINED

Select oils that include the word *unrefined* on the label. They still contain their original vitamins and minerals, chlorophyll, and such compounds as phytoestrogens, which the refining process can destroy or remove. The only widely sold unrefined oil is extra-virgin olive oil; however, you can also find unrefined safflower oil, a polyunsaturated oil, in natural food stores.

Another unrefined oil that deserves to be a staple in your kitchen is flaxseed oil, as it is a very rich source of omega-3 fatty acids. Flaxseed oil is very fragile and will become rancid when exposed to heat, light, or air. For this reason, it is sold in opaque plastic bottles and kept in the refrigerator section in stores. *Never heat flaxseed oil.* Add it to food after the food has been cooked and placed on a serving plate. Or use it in salad dressing, mixed with extra-virgin olive oil. Be sure to make the dressing fresh each time you have some.

BUTTER IS BETTER

While butter is a saturated fat, it is stable and not readily broken down by light, oxygen, or heat. Butter is minimally processed and still contains the natural antioxidants, vitamin E and selenium. The finest quality butter is unsalted and organic.

In contrast, margarine is made from highly refined oil that is heated to high temperatures, generating trans-fatty acids. A trans-fatty acid has an unnatural twist in its structure. In your body, trans-fatty acids can increase blood cholesterol levels and blood fat levels, both risk factors for heart disease. They can also interfere with sugar metabolism, the immune response, and pregnancy, and may even be a factor in cancer.

When to Begin—the Sooner the Better

If you are not yet in menopause or have just begun to notice changes in your body, you can do yourself a big favor by starting to eat well. The number of symptoms you may experience at menopause depends on your state of health when menopause begins. As Russell Jaffee, M.D., points out, "The difficulties women experience at menopause are linked to their nutritional deficiencies, not their chronology."

Closely allied with nutrition is the use of herbs to create health during menopause. Step 3 of the Healthy Menopause Program shows you how to make use of herbs to ease symptoms.

CHAPTER SIX

Step 3: Herbs and Menopause

The Healthy Menopause Program relies for the most part on natural means of healing and achieving well-being. One of the most important aspects of this program is the use of herbs. Many herbs have medicinal effects, just like pharmaceutical drugs, but fundamentally they too are food. Think of them as a source of nourishment just like bananas and pumpkin seeds!

Producers of herbal remedies use raw materials derived from cultivated plants or those collected in the wild. Herbs are not necessarily derived from true herbs. Herbal medicine also makes use of roots, leaves, seeds, and the bark of shrubs, vines, and trees. Some are taken in capsule form like any prescription. Some can be added to everyday meals or enjoyed brewed as teas.

Drugs consist of isolated ingredients. In contrast, medicinal plants contain a variety of healing substances. For this reason, herbalists will often use the whole plant in treating a patient. The seemingly less useful components work synergistically with the active ingredients to deliver a far more gentle form of healing than pharmaceuticals offer. Plants contain two fundamental types of compounds: active ingredients, which chemists study and drug manufacturers research to develop new products; and all the other substances and compounds that are largely ignored by modern medicine. It is the totality of these that herbalists rely on to promote healing and health.

The supporting compounds may help the body more easily benefit from an herb or temper the action of a very potent plant chemical, helping to prevent side effects. Some substances may even prevent overdosing by triggering nausea when an individual has taken more of a plant than the system can tolerate. Herbs can be effective treatments and tonics, thanks to their primary active ingredients as well as these secondary compounds.

Special Compounds

Healing plants and herbs contain a range of health-supportive substances. One category is the *volatile oils,* which include alkaloids, bitters, flavonoids, glycosides, and tannins. Another group is the *steroidal saponins.* These compounds have an effect on the production and balance of hormones that are also steroids. Saponins are present in various herbs used traditionally for female health, such as black cohosh, blue cohosh, ginseng, false unicorn root, squaw vine, fenugreek, wild yam, and licorice.

Drugs have a single effect, whereas herbs have a complexity of actions, which explains why they can be used to treat what can only be considered as opposite conditions. Herbs that contain phytohormones can be used as a remedy for low estrogen as well as low progesterone.

If using herbal medicine seems to you a bit too folksy, even risky, consider this: At least 25% of all modern pharmaceutical drugs are derived from herbs. In addition, the classic herbs used to treat such problems as hot flashes and mood swings have a legacy of success that spans centuries. Native American women relied on black cohosh to balance sex hormones and reduce menopausal symptoms, and this herb is still prescribed for menopause today.

Herbal Remedies Can Be Taken in Many Forms

One option is to buy dried plants and make up your own preparations to save money. You can even buy empty gelatin capsules and fill these yourself with the herbs you plan to take. However, such a hands-on approach takes time and effort and is not recommended for newcomers to herbal medicine. Start with ready-made, high-quality herbal products such as whole herbs, herbal extracts and tinctures, and herbs in capsules.

- You can prepare a cup of healing herbal tea right in your own kitchen by brewing the dried leaves, stems, or flowers of a plant such as mint or chamomile. Put a teaspoon of dried herbs in a teapot and pour a cup of boiling water over them. Then place the cover on the pot and allow the tea to steep for 10 to 15 minutes. Herbalists refer to herbal teas as *infusions*.

  You can also brew tea from a fresh herb such as mint. In this case, use two to three teaspoons of herb per cup. Steep for 10 to 15 minutes. Pour yourself a cup of tea and sit back and relax while your brew gently takes effect. Brewed teas keep for up to 2 days in the refrigerator.

- If you're working with a specialist in traditional Chinese medicine for your menopausal symptoms, you may be given packets of a variety of plant materials that need to be cooked to extract their healing compounds. Such a preparation is called a *decoction*. The herbs are boiled in water for as long as 20 or 30 minutes. The plant material is then strained out, leaving the medicinal liquid. Roots, barks, and seeds, which are hard, are usually prepared in this way, as they require longer exposure to heat in order to extract their active compounds.

- You may decide to take herbs in the form of prepared *tinctures*. Herbs are kept for about 2 weeks in a solution of alcohol and water, both of which act as solvents and dissolve nearly all the relevant ingredients in the plant. The herbs are then removed and the remaining liquid is the tincture. Because a tincture is a liquid, herbs in this form are more easily absorbed. However, tinctures sometimes have a bitter taste.

- You'll find many herbal medicines sold in *tablet* and *capsule* form. This is the most convenient way of taking herbs. However, some women who are already supplementing with a variety of vitamins and minerals decide that they do not want another pill to swallow, and prefer the liquid tinctures and extracts.

Herbs often work best in combination. Various hormone-balancing and menopause formulas can be found in health food stores, shops specializing in herbs, and through mail order. A good formula for menopausal women might contain such herbs as alfalfa, black cohosh, red clover, chasteberry, false unicorn, ginseng, holy thistle, licorice root, sarsaparilla, and squaw vine.

Using Herbs Safely

The medicinal herbs commonly taken today have been used for treating ailments for hundreds if not thousands of years. The herbs that were obviously poisonous have long been removed from the herbal pharmacy. In addition, over the centuries the best ways to take herbs were carefully recorded, as well as any side effects. However, whenever you take herbs, you still need to use caution, as some herbs are dangerous if you have certain medical conditions, if you are taking particular drugs, or if you are pregnant or nursing.

Work with a skilled professional, such as an herbalist or naturopathic physician. Even if you self-prescribe, be sure to check with a specialist who can assess the herbs you plan to take.

In addition, do not exceed recommended dosages. The labels of many herbal products give recommended amounts. These are generally safe to follow. If you have any question about dosage, consult with a trained specialist.

Watching for Side Effects

When taken appropriately, herbs should not cause significant side effects. If side effects do occur, they are usually relatively benign and may include nausea, diarrhea, and skin reactions. However, an individual may experience more serious side effects such as hypertension and allergic reaction. Before taking any herbal preparation, it is essential that you know the signs of toxicity and watch for these. In addition, if you are taking any form of drug or medication, be sure to inform your supervising physician that you plan to take herbs so that a potential drug-herb interaction can be avoided.

Making Sure an Herbal Product Is Reliable, with a Safe Potency

The potency of herbs naturally varies from plant to plant, so one batch of prepared herbs may be less effective at treating a medical problem than another batch. To avoid these differences when buying capsules of prepared herbs, look for products that are "standardized preparations." The manufacturer produces consistent levels of key ingredients in each batch of pills.

Commercial medicinal herbs produced in Europe are usually reliable products. German products, as well as those made in Switzerland, must meet tough governmental standards and are by law standardized preparations.

The U.S. Pharmacopeia, a nonprofit organization, began in 1998 to publish the first American standards for the potency of certain herbs, including chamomile, which may be used to alleviate anxiety and promote sleep. Herbal product manufacturers who observe these standards are permitted to add NF (national formulary) to their labels.

Nonstandardized products are usually made from whole herbs and the potency of these products can vary greatly.

Freshness

Look for an expiration date on the label of the product you are buying. This will give you some idea of the herb's shelf life. Healing oils and other compounds can deteriorate and become ineffective.

Sources of Herbs

Most herbal substances used in North America are imported from other countries. Sources include China, India, many European countries, and South America—locales where herbal medicine has long been practiced. In buying imported herbs, it is important to select reputable brands. Look for herbs that are free of chemicals and preferably raised organically.

Be Sure to Tell Your Physician That You Are Taking Herbs

Even if you are taking herbs under the direction of a skilled herbalist, make certain you also inform your regular physician about the herbs and dosages you are taking. Your doctor needs this information to be on the lookout for side effects and to consider possible interactions between these herbs and any medications that might be prescribed. As many as 15 million Americans take herbs along with prescription medications, but 60% of patients never tell their doctors they are taking herbs.

Call the Manufacturer

If you have a question about the herbal supplements you are taking, you can always speak with a representative of the company that produces them. Here are some questions to ask the manufacturer:

- How long has the company been in business?
- What kind of quality-control programs are in place?
- How are the identity of the herb and its potency determined?
- Is the company a member of any trade groups such as the American Herbal Products Association (AHPA)?

While membership in an association is not a guarantee of quality, AHPA actively promotes self-regulation and is working with the U.S. Food and Drug Administration to implement various mandates of the 1994 Dietary Supplements Health and Education Act.

Starting and Stopping Your Use of Herbs

Remember to incorporate herbs into any regimen of self-care slowly. And if you decide to discontinue taking herbs, also be sure to taper off slowly. Your body will be better able to adjust and you will be less likely to experience side effects.

Use menopause as your opportunity to experience the gentle and healing properties of these natural allies. Thanks to menopause, many women have tried herbs for the first time and discovered their ability to ease menopausal symptoms and enhance health. Now it's your turn.

Incorporating Herbs into an Overall Plan for Self-Care

Herbs can have a gentle but cumulative effect on your health, helping you to enjoy years of well-being and freedom from disease. But herbs are not magic pills. Taking herbs alone cannot do away with symptoms of menopause or ensure long-term health if you are eating a nutrient-poor diet, are not exercising, and are unable to manage everyday stresses and demands. Taking herbs can play a role in bettering your health, but you also need to follow the other recommendations of the Healthy Menopause Program.

A Glossary of Herbs

The following herbs have been found useful in easing the symptoms of menopause. You may find that a single herb is all you need. Some women use a combination of herbs and work with a trained herbalist to adjust their formula until results are achieved. You are the ultimate authority on which herbs, if any, are right for you.

Many of the most commonly prescribed herbs for menopause have an effect on reproductive hormones, either by increasing hormone levels or by balancing hormones. These herbs include dong quai, black cohosh, Siberian ginseng, and red clover. Following is a description of each herb, including benefits, active compounds, suggestions on how to take the herb, and cautions about its use.

Dong Quai

Dong quai is a Chinese herb second only in popularity to ginseng among the Chinese. It is also known as "angelica," from its Latin name, *Angelica sinensis.*

Benefits: This valued medicinal herb has traditionally been used to treat symptoms of menopause such as hot flashes and thinning of vaginal tissue. Dong quai is moisturizing, counteracting reduced vaginal lubrication. Dong quai soothes the entire pelvic area, relieving aches and cramps, and restores vitality and warmth to the tissues. This herb is also routinely prescribed for complaints related to premenstrual syndrome (PMS), which can be associated with perimenopause. Dong quai is useful in treating depression. This herb also helps regulate the menstrual cycle, which can become irregular during perimenopause.

Dong quai enhances blood flow to the skin and can bring a glow to the complexion, and it is used to help smooth out fine lines and thicken skin that has thinned with age. Dong quai can also help thicken vaginal walls. In addition, this herb protects the cardiovascular system, helping prevent heart disease, which women are more vulnerable to as they age.

How it works: The benefits of dong quai are thought to be due to the mild estrogenic effect of the herb and to active compounds that help stabilize blood vessels.

Taking dong quai: As an infusion, take ½ to 1 cup daily. As a tincture, take 15 to 30 drops one to three times a day.

Caution: Dong quai is not recommended for women who regularly have bloating, menorrhagia (heavy bleeding), which can occur during perimenopause, or diarrhea. The herb is also not recommended for women with fibroids or those who experience any tenderness or discomfort of the breasts. In addition, dong quai should not be taken by individuals using blood-thinning medications or aspirin.

In terms of Chinese medicine, dong quai is considered a warming herb, particularly beneficial for women who have a constitution that is "low energy" and who tend to feel cold. In contrast, dong quai is not considered appropriate for those with a "high-energy" constitution who tend to feel warm.

Black Cohosh

The use of black cohosh in America dates back centuries when Native Americans and then European colonists relied on this healing herb to treat a variety of complaints. Black cohosh, also known as snake root and squaw root, was a Native American remedy for disorders of the womb, to soothe irritation and congestion in the cervix, womb, and vagina, to ease childbirth, and to promote and restore healthy menstruation.

At the end of the 19th century, physicians considered black cohosh a highly trustworthy remedy for menstrual cramps and prescribed it routinely. The plant grows to 3 feet or more and has white flowers. The medicinal compounds that black cohosh supplies are present in the root of the plant. Its Latin name is *Cimicifuga racemosa.*

Benefits: Black cohosh can benefit the system in three ways. Its active ingredients function as a tonic for the nerves, counteract muscle spasms, and help balance hormones. When used regularly over several months, black cohosh supports the body in producing the hormones it needs to rebalance itself.

Clinical studies investigating the ability of black cohosh to treat menopausal symptoms have shown that this healing herb helps prevent hot flashes and night sweats. Thinning of vaginal tissue and loss of libido are less likely to occur. It is also prescribed to ease aches and pains.

Black cohosh eases the emotional symptoms some women experience, including anxiety, nervousness, and depression. Many health care professionals consider black cohosh a safe and effective alternative to hormone replacement therapy.

How it works: With menopause, the amount of estrogen produced by the ovaries is greatly reduced. In response, the pituitary gland, located in the brain, produces two hormones that stimulate the ovaries to increase estrogen production: luteinizing hormone (LH) and follicle-stimulating hormone (FSH). Elevated levels of luteinizing hormone in particular may trigger symptoms of menopause. Black cohosh has been shown to lower levels of luteinizing hormone. In addition, black cohosh mimics estriol, a type of estrogen that has an anticancer effect.

Taking black cohosh: The herb is sold in a standardized dosage under the brand name Remifemin. This standardized preparation is produced in Germany. Since 1956, over 1.5 million women in Germany have used black cohosh with great success and without significant side effects. Black cohosh is also widely used in Austria and Scandinavia. You can find standardized tablets of black cohosh in North American health food stores and pharmacies.

You can also prepare a decoction. Boil 1 teaspoon of the dried root in a cup of filtered water for 12 minutes. Cool and take a spoonful of the black cohosh tea every few hours during the day. And if you take black cohosh as a tincture of the fresh root, take 10 to 30 drops in a little filtered water sipped throughout the day.

Caution: Black cohosh should not be taken by pregnant women or women experiencing heavy menstrual bleeding. Overdosing can lead to nausea, vomiting, headache, dizziness, limb pain, and lowered blood pressure.

Ginseng and Siberian Ginseng

Ginseng is not one herb but three: Chinese or Korean ginseng, American ginseng, and Siberian ginseng. Ginseng is considered an adaptogen, which covers a broad range of benefits, from stimulating the immune system and counteracting fatigue to helping to prevent heart disease.

ORIENTAL GINSENG OR PANAX GINSENG

This form of ginseng is widely cultivated and is more potent than its American cousin. It is effective in treating very severe symptoms of menopause, especially by increasing stress toler-ance. Stress can bring on and worsen symptoms of menopause (see Chapter 8). Ginseng strengthens the adrenal glands, which are involved in the stress response, and supports the functioning of such glands as the thyroid, pituitary, and hypo-thalamus, which are also sensitive to stress.

Benefits: Oriental ginseng lessens the severity of meno-pausal symptoms and helps relieve the heavy menstrual bleed-ing that can occur during perimenopause.

How it works: Panax ginseng contains ginsenosides, active compounds that have an estrogenic effect and help bal-ance hormones by encouraging the body to produce the mix of hormones needed.

Taking Oriental ginseng: See page 113.

Caution: Panax ginseng is generally considered safe. Massive overdoses can cause sleeplessness, excessive muscle tension (hypertonia), and edema.

Siberian Ginseng

This herb, known as *Eleutherococcus senticosus,* is not a true gin-seng such as Chinese or Korean ginseng, but contains similar active ingredients. Herbalists consider Siberan ginseng more female oriented than its botanical cousins.

Benefits: Siberian ginseng is often included in herbal for-mulas for female health because it enhances the effects of the other herbs in the formula. Siberian ginseng also helps the body respond to stress, which can trigger hot flashes and irri-tability.

How it works: The hypothalamus plays a role in mecha-nisms that bring on hot flashes. Siberian ginseng is thought to influence the hypothalamus by modulating the release of cer-tain hormones.

In addition, components in Siberian ginseng can be converted into stress hormones such as cortisol. Under stress the adrenal glands normally produce such hormones, but with plant-derived hormones present in the system, activation of the adrenal glands and production of cortisol is reduced. The adrenals are spared and are not as likely to become overworked and to worsen menopausal symptoms.

Taking ginseng: Buy ginseng from a reputable source to make sure you take a quality product, to avoid the many relatively low-potency ginseng products on the market. Ginseng can be pricey, but buy the best you can afford. Ginseng is sold in capsule form, as a fresh root tincture and as a powder or cut root for making tea.

As a fresh root tincture, take 5 to 25 drops one to three times a day. As a decoction, brew 1 ounce of root in a cup of hot filtered water. Take ginseng for 6 to 8 weeks for full benefits, as the effects of this herb are cumulative.

Red Clover

Red clover is an invaluable and potent estrogenic plant for treating menopause. It also acts as a mild diuretic, stimulating the body to shed fluids. However, red clover is less commonly prescribed than other estrogenic herbs.

Benefits: Red clover can be useful in reducing hot flashes, relieving insomnia, and improving mood. In one double-blind study, 86 perimenopausal women were given either a red clover supplement supplying 40 milligrams of isoflavones per 500-milligram tablet, or a placebo. The women recorded their symptoms weekly, over 8 months. In addition, levels of isoflavones in urine were measured at the end of the study. The results showed a high correlation between intake of isoflavones from red clover and a reduction of hot flashes.

Red clover also appears to benefit the cardiovascular system. It has been shown to increase blood levels of the desirable form of cholesterol, HDL, as well as relaxing arterial walls, thereby reducing the risk of high blood pressure.

How it works: Like beans and lentils, red clover contains isoflavones, compounds with hormone-like activity. Soybeans in particular have been in the spotlight for their isoflavone content and their usefulness in treating symptoms of menopause. However, red clover deserves a closer look at its potential for supporting female health.

While soy contains two types of isoflavones, daidzein and genistein, red clover contains all four main estrogenic isoflavones: the two just mentioned, plus biochanin and for-mononetin. Giving red clover to patients results in high levels of daidzein and genistein in the blood, moderate levels of biochanin, and low levels of formononetin. Vegetarians who regularly eat legumes, and in general have less difficulty with menopause, have a similar blood profile.

There are several advantages to using red clover as a source of isoflavones rather than soy. Red clover is more potent than soybeans. The plant contains about 2 percent by dry weight of isoflavones, 10 times the percent in soybeans. A woman may need to take only a small amount to experience benefits. In addition, using red clover as a source of isoflavones does not require a change in diet, and unlike soy, red clover does not interfere with the body's ability to extract nourishment from food. Soybeans contain antinutritive factors (see Chapter 5).

Taking red clover: You can buy red clover in pill form, providing a standardized dosage of isoflavones. Two 500-milligram capsules three times a day are recommended.

Another option is to take red clover as a tea, but in this form you have no guarantee of how much isoflavone you are receiving. To make the tea, pour a cup of boiling water over 1 to 3 teaspoonfuls of the dried herb and leave to infuse for 10 to 15 minutes. Have a cup three times a day. Or take red clover as a tincture, ½ teaspoon three times a day.

Read labels carefully. You need to check whether the isoflavones are in their free form or glycoside form—that is, attached to a large sugar molecule. The glycoside form is less potent. Taking 10 milligrams of isoflavones as glycosides is equivalent to taking only 4 milligrams of active, free isoflavones. An average recommended dosage is 40 milligrams a day of isoflavones.

In shopping for red clover, also look for products that are made from the leaves where the active compounds are mostly found. Red clover flowers have only low levels of isoflavones.

Store red clover in a cool, dry place, below 85°F, or in the refrigerator if the climate is hot and humid.

Caution: Red clover is generally considered safe.

More Herbs for Menopause

Chamomile

Chamomile has been used medicinally since Egyptian times. As part of European herbal medicine it was considered a cure-all, renowned for its many medical and household uses.

Benefits: Chamomile lessens anxiety and promotes much needed sleep that may have been lost because of night sweats.

How it works: Chamomile contains many active compounds, including flavonoids and essential oils. It acts as a tonic to the nervous system.

Taking chamomile: To make chamomile tea, use 2 to 3 heaping teaspoons of flowers per cup of boiling water. Steep 10 to 20 minutes. Drink up to 3 cups a day. As a tincture, use ½ to 1 teaspoon up to three times a day.

For a relaxing herbal bath, tie a handful of chamomile flowers into a cloth. Hang this over the faucet and run the bath water through it.

Caution: Chamomile is generally considered safe.

Chasteberry

As its name implies, chasteberry has often been used as a means of lowering sexual desire and libido. Actually, according to modern research, chasteberry normalizes sex drive, suppressing or enhancing libido, whichever is needed. It is also known as vitex for its Latin name, *Vitex agnus-castus*.

Benefits: Chasteberry is recommended to reduce hot flashes and moisten dry vaginal tissues. This herb is also effective in treating problems associated with the PMS-like symptoms of perimenopause: menstrual cramps, bloating, breast tenderness, acne, migraine headaches, and depression. Chasteberry helps regulate the menstrual cycle, which may become irregular at this time.

How it works: Chasteberry is considered a tonic for the reproductive organs. Chasteberry's active ingredients include glycosides and flavonoids. This healing herb acts on the pituitary gland, and may alter luteinizing hormone and follicle-stimulating hormone secreted by this gland. This in turn stimulates production of progesterone.

Taking chasteberry: Chasteberry is a gentle herb. You may need to take it for several months before benefits will be evident. Take chasteberry in capsule form or as a tea. Pour a cup of boiling water over 1 teaspoon of the ripe berries and leave to infuse for 10 to 15 minutes. Drink this three times a day. As a tincture, take 1 to 2 milliliters three times a day.

Caution: Women who are pregnant or nursing mothers should not take chasteberry. In addition, chasteberry occasionally causes rashes. Chasteberry can also interact with dopamine-receptor antagonists, weakening their effect.

False Unicorn Root

This herb was an important part of the herbal pharmacopeia of the North American Indians. Herbalists consider it an outstanding tonic, strengthening the reproductive system in both men and women.

Benefits: This healing herb normalizes reproductive function, helping to balance a woman's own supply of hormones. False unicorn root is able to aid apparently opposite conditions. It can help regulate the menstrual cycle, which can become irregular during perimenopause, and is useful in minimizing symptoms due to dramatic fluctuations in hormone levels.

How it works: False unicorn root contains steroidal saponins, compounds that are precursors to estrogen.

Taking false unicorn root: For a decoction, put 1 to 2 teaspoonfuls of the root in a cup of filtered water, bring to a boil, and simmer gently for 10 to 15 minutes. Drink this three times a day. As a tincture, take 2 to 4 milliliters three times a day. False unicorn root is also available in capsules.

Caution: False unicorn root is generally considered safe; however, in large doses the herb can cause nausea and vomiting.

Gingko Biloba

Gingko biloba is one of the oldest living tree species, with a lineage tracing back more than 200 million years. The tree can grow to 120 feet in height and has a 2-inch leaf with a distinctive fan shape.

In Germany and France, gingko biloba is among the leading prescription medicines. In North America, it is classed as a food supplement and sold in standardized dosages. Gingko biloba's safety is well established.

Benefits: Dozens of studies show that individuals taking gingko biloba experience improved mental performance. For women in menopause, gingko biloba improves short-term memory as well as countering fatigue and nervousness caused by an inadequate supply of oxygen and blood sugar to body tissues. The herb is also prescribed for vertigo, tinnitus (ringing in the ears), and depression.

How it works: The brain has only small reserves of energy and requires a continuous supply of large amounts of both oxygen and glucose to be delivered by the blood to brain tissue. An extract taken from the gingko leaves is used medicinally to improve blood flow to the brain, and to enhance the use of oxygen and glucose by increasing cellular intake.

Taking gingko biloba: A standardized dosage is 40 milligrams, three times a day, of the extract standardized to contain 24% glycosides and 6% terpene lactones. Gingko is commonly taken in capsule form.

Caution: Gingko biloba is generally considered safe, but in rare instances side effects can include intestinal problems, headaches, and dizziness. Overdosing can lead to irritability, restlessness, diarrhea, and vomiting. Gingko is a blood thinner and should not be taken along with blood-thinning medications such as aspirin and warfarin (Coumadin).

Licorice

Licorice is prescribed to treat a range of complaints including arthritis, inflammation, bacterial infection, asthma, and high cholesterol. Licorice also has a marked effect on the endocrine system and helps support normal functioning of the adrenal glands and reproductive system. Most licorice candy on the market does not contain licorice and is flavored with fennel instead. However, many imported brands are made with the actual herb.

Benefits: Licorice supports the adrenal glands, which can have an impact on menopause. The adrenals are a source of estrogen precursors postmenopause and also help buffer stress, which can worsen menopausal symptoms.

How it works: Glycyrrhizin, the active compound in

licorice, helps to maintain normal levels of progesterone and cortisol by suppressing the primary enzyme responsible for inactivating these. Isoflavonoids and glycyrrhetinic acid, a compound released when glycyrrhizin is broken down, help balance the body's estrogen level. This action in particular works to reduce the PMS-like symptoms of perimenopause that are caused by high estrogen levels relative to progesterone.

Taking licorice: As a decoction, put ½ to 1 teaspoonful of the root in a cup of water, bring to a boil, and simmer for 10 to 15 minutes. Drink this three times a day. As a tincture, take 1 to 3 milliliters of the tincture three times a day.

Caution: Large doses of licorice taken over a long period of time can lead to high blood pressure, water retention, and high sodium and low potassium levels in the blood. Licorice is not appropriate if you have a history of hypertension, diabetes, glaucoma, stroke, or heart attack. In addition, pregnant and nursing women should not take licorice.

Motherwort

Motherwort has a place in the Chinese pharmacopoeia. It has been traditionally used as a sedative, calming the nervous system while acting as a tonic to the whole body.

Benefits: Motherwort can lessen symptoms of anxiety associated with menopause and can ease hot flashes, which can be brought on by stress. This herb can reduce their intensity, length, and frequency. Motherwort also promotes sleep, helping counteract menopausal fatigue caused by night sweats.

The herb helps restore elasticity of the vaginal walls by improving circulation and thickening tissues. In addition, motherwort lessens PMS-like symptoms that may occur during perimenopause. It functions as a diuretic, reducing fluid retention, and also helps prevent menstrual cramps when menstrual flow is light, moderate, or absent.

How it works: Motherwort is rich in natural compounds that act as a mild sedative, prevent muscle spasms, regulate the heart, and stimulate and promote normal menstrual flow.

Taking motherwort: Motherwort, which has a bitter taste, is most palatable taken as a tincture. Take ⅛ to ¾ teaspoon of the tincture three times a day. As a tea, pour a cup of boiling water over 1 to 2 teaspoonfuls of the dried herb and leave to infuse for 10 to 15 minutes. Drink this three times a day. Motherwort is also available in capsules.

Caution: The herb is not recommended for women with excessive menstrual flow, which can occur during perimenopause, as motherwort can increase menstrual flow. Also, as with all herbs, consult your doctor before taking it if you are pregnant or lactating.

Garden Sage

This common culinary herb has been found to have some estrogen-like activity. (Fennel and anise also contain estrogenic compounds.) You can easily grow garden sage, *Salvia officianalis*, in your own backyard or in a flower pot, but don't plan on harvesting "sage" growing wild in the desert. That sage is a different plant, called dessert sage or sagebrush.

Benefits: Sage helps balance hormones and has been used since ancient Roman times to treat PMS, increase fertility, and ease the transition to menopause. Sage also helps quell hot flashes and night sweats. This herb soothes nerves and helps prevent headaches.

How it works: During perimenopause, the tannins and volatile oils in sage help limit excessive menstrual flow that can occur as hormone levels become erratic. In addition, this ancient herb is rich in minerals such as potassium and magnesium, which tend to be excreted from the body in perspiration that usually follows a hot flash.

Taking garden sage: Take sage as a tea: pour a cup of boiling water over 1 to 2 teaspoonfuls of the leaves and let infuse for 10 minutes. Drink three times a day, or before retiring, to reduce night sweats. As a tincture, take 2 to 4 milliliters of the tincture three times a day.

Caution: This herb is generally considered safe. However, sage is better suited to perimenopause than menopause itself. As sage is a drying herb, it is not an appropriate herb for women troubled by vaginal dryness. Since sage stimulates the muscles of the uterus, it should be avoided during pregnancy.

Sarsaparilla

Sarsaparilla (*Smilax officinalis*) is valued for its root and rhizome. In general, this herb has been prescribed traditionally to restore proper functioning of all body systems, including the endocrine system, which produces hormones, and to enliven the body as a whole. Yes, sarsaparilla is also a beverage, a carbonated drink that was very popular in the mid-1800s. Sarsaparilla drink on the market today is flavored artificially, not with the beneficial herb.

Benefits: Sarsaparilla is frequently added to general herbal formulas for menopause to normalize the rhythm of the menstrual cycle during perimenopause, and to increase sex drive.

How it works: Sarsaparilla contains hormone-like compounds and is used traditionally to support progesterone production. It also contains compounds with properties that aid the activity of testosterone, the hormone that fuels libido.

Taking sarsaparilla: To make a decoction, put 1 to 2 teaspoonfuls of the root in a cup of filtered water, bring to a boil, and simmer for 10 to 15 minutes. Drink this three times a day. As a tincture, take ⅛ to ¼ teaspoon three times a day. Sarsaparilla is also available in capsules.

Caution: In rare cases, taking sarsaparilla can cause stomach upset and queasiness, as well as kidney irritation. Overdosing can lead to various serious conditions including excessive urination, European cholera, and shock.

Valerian

Valerian is a perennial plant native to North America and Europe, and can reach 2 to 4 feet in height. The root is used medicinally.

Benefits: Like chamomile, valerian can ease tension and anxiety, as well as promote restful sleep. Valerian is more potent than chamomile.

How it works: Two active compounds found exclusively in valerian, valepotriates and valeric acid, are responsible for the sedative effect of this herb.

Taking valerian: As a mild sedative, use a standard extract with 0.8% valeric acid content. The standard dosage is 150 to 300 milligrams, taken 30 to 45 minutes before bedtime.

Caution: Valerian is generally considered safe, although in rare cases, intestinal problems can occur.

A QUICK LOOK AT HERBS FOR MENOPAUSE

Hot Flashes, Night Sweats
dong quai

black cohosh

Siberian ginseng

red clover

chasteberry

licorice

false unicorn root

motherwort

sage

Fatigue

Panax ginseng

motherwort

gingko biloba

chamomile

valerian

ginger

Mood Swings

black cohosh

Panax ginseng

red clover

sarsaparilla

licorice

false unicorn root

gingko biloba

Anxiety, Irritability

Panax ginseng

Siberian ginseng

black cohosh

red clover

motherwort

chamomile

valerian

licorice

sage

Depression
dong quai
chasteberry
gingko biloba

Poor Memory
gingko biloba

Thinning Vaginal Tissue
dong quai
black cohosh
motherwort

Vaginal Dryness
dong quai
chasteberry
gingko biloba

Sexual Desire
black cohosh
chasteberry
sarsaparilla

Menstrual Cramps
dong quai
black cohosh
chasteberry
motherwort

Heavy Menstrual Bleeding
Panax ginseng

sage

red clover

Irregular Menstrual Cycle
chasteberry

dong quai

sarsaparilla

false unicorn root

Fluid Retention
red clover

chasteberry

motherwort

CHAPTER SEVEN

Step 4: Exercise and Menopause

The fourth step in the Healthy Menopause Program is exercise. Physical activity feels good because it is good for you! Movement benefits the body, the mind, and the spirit. Children instinctively know this and relish being physically active. Unfortunately, many adults seem to have forgotten the pure pleasure of moving their bodies.

Exercise benefits female health in several ways. Physical movement increases circulation of the blood, allowing more nutrients to reach target tissues and cells. Exercise stretches stiff tendons and makes them more supple. Physical activity causes more oxygen to reach the brain, stimulating mental function. A good workout dispels stress, a known trigger for menopausal symptoms, and exercise can help maintain a normal weight. Being overweight in itself can lead to hormone imbalances and related menopausal problems.

It is no wonder many women are finding that regular exercise can help reduce symptoms of menopause and that exercise needs to be a component of any overall plan of self-care. Hot flashes, irritability, sleeplessness, fatigue, and memory can all be improved with physical activity. In addition, exercise can help lower the risk of degenerative disease, including osteoporosis and heart disease, which women are more prone to as they age.

Ancient and Modern Forms of Exercise

Certain types of exercise are particularly effective in keeping women well. There are those that involve slow movement, controlled breathing, and even meditative thought. These include yoga, tai chi, and qigong (pronounced "chee kung"). These disciplines, all three originating in Eastern cultures, developed over centuries and consist of a variety of postures and choreographed movements that target specific components of the anatomy. Certain poses in particular nourish female health. These practices can leave you feeling wonderfully vitalized after a single session. However, consistent practice over many months brings even greater benefits, healing the body and building a foundation for good health.

But women at midlife also need active, vigorous physical activity that can stimulate the system and support the healthy functioning of organs, tissues, and cells. Jogging, aerobics, and weight-bearing exercise are prime examples of the modern and Westernized approach to exercise. These can help temper signs of menopause and also exercise the heart and strengthen bones.

Sometimes the walk from the sofa to the front door is the most difficult exercise of all. Make up your mind to give yourself the gift of exercise. If you want inspiration, remember how good it can feel to stretch your legs and draw in fresh air. Remember the exhilaration you feel after exercising, how clear your mind is and free of worries. Take a walk right now!

Getting Started

You may be thinking that you hate jogging and you'll never be caught in an aerobics class with a bunch of 20-somethings. But don't let this stop you from exercising altogether. If you don't already exercise, the first step is simply to begin, and it doesn't matter how.

Start with a walk through the mall. If you want company, you may even be able to join a mall-walking group. These are cropping up in cities that are subject to exceptionally cold or hot weather, where residents are in need of indoor exercise space away from the elements. Members window-shop and chat while exercising!

Tackle a creative home project that you've been wanting to do, perhaps some landscaping. Or buy a gallon of paint and give a wall in your home a new lease on life. Such projects will have you moving muscles you didn't know were there.

Live out a fantasy. Take that tap dancing class you've always thought about. If you can't keep your feet from moving while you watch a Fred Astaire movie, perhaps ballroom dancing is for you. Have you always wanted an adventure vacation rather than sitting at the beach? Contact environmentalist groups or ask around at your local science museum or university for opportunities to do some field work as a volunteer. Tagging turtles, sifting through sand, or cleaning up the environment in some way can get you moving!

The following sections take a closer look at certain types of exercise that have been found to be good for women and may be just what you need too.

Yoga for Women

Yoga is an ancient practice, developed in India thousands of years ago, and yoga continues today to be a powerful and effective way of maintaining health. Take advantage of yogic wisdom to facilitate your passage through perimenopause and into menopause. Yoga is a form of exercise, a meditative discipline, and also a means of becoming at peace with yourself. As Robert Birnberg, a yoga instructor based in Los Angeles, explains, "Menopause can be confronting to women who see this as a sign that their youth is over and that they are no longer of use in the society. But yoga offers women a way to accept and be comfortable with the changes that menopause brings and to experience menopause from a new perspective. Yoga postures and breathing techniques can help a woman establish a healthy relationship with herself. And yoga draws a person's attention inward, rather than to outside problems, which with time, can feel less of a burden."

The physical moves of yoga consist of two parts: disciplined breathing and the postures. These poses are held for a given length of time, measured in breaths. You can perform yoga at virtually any age, because yoga offers a variety of exercises and routines that can be tailored to any level of physical ability. Even women in wheelchairs do yoga.

Yogic Breathing

A primary focus of yoga is to enhance the benefits of breathing, the taking in of oxygen, which will bring life to the cells, and the expelling of carbon dioxide, a toxin that must be removed from the body. If you are like most people, your breathing is shallow. Your body barely moves as you inhale and exhale. Yogic breathing is deep and full. On an inhale, the chest expands. On an exhale, the abdomen pulls in, moving the air out through the lungs.

There is research that following a regular pattern of breathing can control hot flashes. In a 1992 study published in the *American Journal of Obstetrics and Gynecology*, researchers experimented with paced breathing to reduce hot flashes. Thirty-three women who were experiencing frequent hot flashes were asked to slow their breathing. By doing so, they were able to significantly reduce the frequency of hot flashes. The researchers suggested that such an approach to managing hot flashes could be especially useful for women who cannot tolerate hormone replacement therapy.

Try the following if you feel a hot flash coming on. Slow your breathing and take only five or six breaths a minute, about one every 10 seconds. You may want to practice doing this in advance, counting slowly from 1 to 5 for each inhalation and from 1 to 5 for each exhalation. As you slow down your breathing, you may actually be able to stop your hot flash in mid-course.

Rhythmic, deep breathing also calms the mind and smoothes emotions. The mood swings and irritability that may occur during perimenopause can be tempered by modulated breathing.

Yoga Postures for Menopause

Yoga postures evolved as a way of facilitating and enhancing this way of breathing. A posture may involve opening the arms wide and pressing them back. This opens the chest. The following move might be a bend from the waist, which automatically compresses the abdomen and physically initiates an exhale.

Yoga poses stimulate circulation, massage and tone the organs and inner muscles, and keep the body limber—a proven way to ensure youthful aging. It's not hard to find yoga teachers in their 60s and 70s. Some women begin taking yoga classes in their 80s. Practicing yoga also helps balance the endocrine system, evening out the glandular and hormonal changes that occur at menopause.

What about twisting your body into pretzel shapes? This is the mental picture most people have in their minds when they think of yoga. These advanced postures are for the experts, but you don't need to do these in order to benefit from yoga. In fact, trying to do overly difficult poses can get in your way. In the world of yoga, struggle is not associated with success, and the motto is not "just do it!" The yoga exercises that will help most with menopausal symptoms are those that you can do while keeping your breathing full and steady, without straining to the point of feeling pain.

Some of the most beneficial yoga postures for menopause are described here. As you read through these, you may want to try some of the suggested positions, but resist the temptation. To make sure you don't put too much strain on a muscle or twist your back, take the time to first find a yoga teacher who can show you how to perform these moves safely. Ideally, have a private lesson and work out a series of postures, selected from the ones in this chapter, suited to your ability and needs. Start with a few simple ones that you can commit to performing on a regular basis, and add more difficult poses only after the first ones begin to seem easy.

INVERSIONS

Yoga postures that involve inverting the body have long been valued for their cooling effect and are known to reduce hot flashes. They also quiet brain activity. If you want to begin with a very simple posture, lie on your back with your buttocks close to a wall and your legs raised and resting on the wall. Stay in this position for 5 or 10 minutes, taking long, even breaths and keeping your eyes closed.

Next you may want to try the Supported Half Shoulderstand (Viparita Karani) and the Full Shoulderstand (Sarvangasana). However, to reduce the risk of injuring yourself, you need to first experiment with these poses with the help of a yoga teacher. Headstands and handstands are the most advanced of the inversion postures.

These positions affect the flow of blood to every organ in the body, including the glands of the endocrine system. Certain positions tend to normalize the function of these glands, helping prevent hormone fluctuations, which can trigger hot flashes. When the body is inverted, the venous blood, which is cooler, drains out of the legs and into the pelvic area and abdomen, helping to prevent the body from heating up.

An inverted posture also helps lower elevated blood pressure and reduces fluid retention, which can occur during perimenopause. This comes about as the pose sends the body a signal that blood pressure has increased. In response, the body quickly takes steps to reduce blood pressure. Blood vessels relax, and excess fluids and salt, which can increase blood pressure, are excreted.

Yoga is also thought to affect the life force within the body, known as *prana*. Inverting the body is said to draw the life force inward, toward the organs, and away from the skin where heating occurs during a hot flash.

FORWARD BENDS

Forward bends are especially soothing and calming both to the nervous system and the mind. These movements gently stretch the spine, promote relaxation, and reduce mood swings and anxiety. Examples include the Head to Knee Pose (Janu Sirsasana) and the Standing Forward Bend Pose (Uttanasana). Yoga teachers sometimes recommend these poses to clear up a case of the blues. Forward bends are also a symbolic way of expressing acceptance of the natural changes occurring.

A forward bend places gentle pressure on the abdominal area, including the uterus and ovaries, and squeezes the blood from these tissues. When you raise your body and come out of the pose, freshly oxygenated blood bathes these organs and enhances their function.

TWISTS

After menopause, your body begins to produce a significant amount of estrogen via the adrenals. The kidneys also become involved. Yoga poses that require twisting are especially good for stimulating these organs. Examples include the Half Fish Pose, which can be done on the floor or sitting in a chair. The idea is to twist the torso so that you are looking over your shoulder. This twist involves more than just the spine and comes from deep within the body.

Another type of pose that stimulates the adrenals and kidneys but takes more agility than a basic twist is the Bow Pose (Dhanurasana), which looks like its name. You begin by lying on your belly, bending your knees, and reaching for your ankles, which you then grip with your hands and hold for 5 to 10 breaths.

These positions stimulate the functioning of the kidneys and adrenals, including the production of estrogen.

WEIGHT-BEARING POSES

Poses that put extra force on your legs and arms help strengthen your bones. The Half Dog Pose and the Downward-Facing Dog Pose (Adho Mukha Svanasana) achieve this. The Half Dog can be done by placing the palms of the hands against the wall, fingers leading upward at chest height. You then step back until your torso is parallel to the floor and your legs are at right angles to the floor. Your body, the wall, and the floor together form a square. In the Full Dog Pose, you bend over with buttocks raised and form a triangle with the floor.

Weight-bearing yogic exercises draw minerals to the bones and stimulate bones to thicken. Yoga also builds muscle and enhances a sense of balance, which can help prevent falls and related bone fractures.

ACTIVELY RELAXING

Relaxing muscles can relieve aches and pains, reduce fatigue, and improve the quality of sleep. This posture is guaranteed to relax you. Lie on your back, a pose known appropriately as the Corpse Pose (Savasana). Close your eyes. Relax your neck muscles and look for any other tension throughout your body. Sink into the earth. Quiet your breathing and your thoughts and remain this way for 10 minutes. Just focus on the ebb and flow of your breath. When you are finished, roll your body to one side and slowly sit up. This posture is performed at the end of every yoga practice but also works on its own as a substitute for a quick nap.

Giving yourself this downtime strengthens and soothes the sympathetic nervous system, which helps you to manage stress. Becoming peaceful is also known to reduce high blood pressure.

SUBTLE MOVEMENTS

This yoga pose (Aswini Mudra) works the vaginal muscles and the sphincter muscles of the anus, and is similar to the well-known Kegel exercise. Aswini Mudra helps prevent incontinence and the need to urinate more frequently, which can begin to develop at menopause. This pose also helps prevent vaginal infection and dryness. Sit tall, in a comfortable position, with the spine lengthened. Contract the vaginal and sphincter muscles as if you are trying to keep from urinating. Hold this pose for a few breaths and then relax the pose for a few breaths. Repeat 5 to 10 times, extending the length of each contract and relaxation as you become more comfortable with the pose.

This pose increases blood flow to the pelvic area and tones pelvic muscles in the pelvic floor area.

Qigong

Qigong was developed in China more than 500 years ago, and, like yoga, is a time-honored form of exercise that uses movement and breath for healing. A premise of Chinese medicine is that health is a function of Qi (pronounced "chee"), which means vital energy, life force, or life energy, which must continue to flow within the body in order to maintain health and sustain life. In qigong, movement, breath, and mental focus keep that energy moving and increase chi if it is deficient.

In terms of menopause, qigong helps normalize the production of hormones and facilitates the delivery of oxygen and nutrients to the cells, which in turn can ease this transition. When stress begins to overtake you, use qigong as a form of natural first-aid. Lengthening and deepening the breath, slowing movements, and calming the mind can come to your rescue whenever you find yourself in a stressful situation.

Tai Chi

Tai chi is a form of qigong and benefits the female body in the same way. Methodical, slow movements are coupled with controlled breathing and conscious relaxation, merging the physical and the mental. Tai chi, a means of stress management, can ease the symptoms of menopause. In addition, using tai chi faithfully can help reduce the risk of osteoporosis. The movements are weight-bearing exercises that naturally make bones stronger, and the positions also help develop muscle coordination and balance. A woman trained in tai chi may be less likely to take a fall that could result in a bone fracture.

Compared with qigong, tai chi takes longer to learn, but

practicing tai chi over time can pay off. The Chinese use the practice of tai chi as a form of old-age health insurance and you can too.

Begin with Lessons

You might be able to pick up some of the basics of qigong and tai chi in a book or through videotapes, but you'll be learning the hard way and even risking injury. It is far better to take some lessons from an accomplished instructor who will select certain moves especially suited to your capability and needs. You can then do these exercises at home; however, you'll still want to check in from time to time with your teacher for a review and possibly some changes to your routine. In these disciplines, even teachers continue to receive training from their teachers.

Weight-Bearing, Low-Impact, Aerobic Exercise

You need to give yourself some aerobic and weight-bearing exercise each week to make sure that both your heart and bones are benefiting. You may choose to walk in your neighborhood or through city streets on your lunch hour and go to the gym twice a week to lift some weights. Or you can give yourself both types of exercise at the same time by attaching weights made for this purpose to your ankles and wrists, or dancing while holding weights in each hand. The minimum recommendation is three exercise sessions a week, each lasting 20 minutes. But for best results, many researchers advocate exercising for longer periods of time, from 30 to 60 minutes, three to four times a week. Try to exercise hard enough to break a sweat. Each facet of weight-bearing, low-impact aerobic exercise provides special benefits.

Benefits of Aerobic Exercise

The point of aerobic exercise is to speed up your heart rate and your rate of breathing. It includes such activities as running up stairs, walking briskly, waltzing, swimming, and cross-country skiing. This form of activity brings oxygen into your system and stimulates blood circulation, which is important for health at any time, including menopause. Better circulation in the pelvic area may help relieve changes in vaginal tissue. Increased blood flow allows more oxygen and glucose to reach brain tissue. Improved circulation clears the mind of brain fog that can show up as hormone production declines. This sort of energetic activity is also a good way to relieve tension and stress, which can worsen such menopausal symptoms as hot flashes, irritability, and fatigue. And if you are troubled by night sweats and have disturbed sleep, feeling tired from vigorous exercise may help you return to sleep more quickly. Even taking a purposeful but unhurried walk regularly, at the same time each day, can be calming and help symptoms.

Aerobic exercise is excellent for heart health. According to the American Heart Association, regularly doing this sort of exercise lowers cholesterol levels and blood pressure. It improves the survival rate of individuals who have already had a heart attack and reduces the likelihood of their suffering a second one. Even modest levels of physical activity can be beneficial. Walking is an integral part of the lifestyle program, developed by Dean Ornish, M.D., that has been proven to reverse heart disease after a period of a year. Participants in the program are also asked to reduce fat intake to 10% and to follow a diet of unrefined, unprocessed foods, to receive stress management training, and to stop smoking.

Benefits of Low-Impact Aerobics

Low-impact aerobic exercise involves quick steps, skips, and gentle dance steps, performed with speed over a length of time, to give the heart a workout. When done properly, low-impact aerobics are gentle on tissues and joints. In contrast, high-impact aerobics involves leaps, hard landings, and jumping jacks. Particularly if you have not exercised for a while, this rough exercise can strain muscles and damage joints. High-impact aerobics also puts stress on the tissue in the abdominal area where your reproductive organs are located. If you do not have a strong girdle of abdominal muscles for protection, you need to temper your exercise. In fact, well-planned aerobics of either sort should begin with a few easy sit-ups so that you are more conscious of this part of your anatomy and remember to use these muscles as you exercise other parts of your body.

You needn't join an exercise class to include low-impact aerobics in your everyday life. Just walking down the street qualifies as low-impact. Enjoying a night of ballroom dancing also qualifies, as does playing golf if you walk the whole course.

Benefits of Weight-Bearing Exercise

Weight-bearing exercise is recommended for women because it strengthens bones, thereby reducing the risk of osteoporosis. This form of exercise actually triggers bone building due to the *piezoelectric effect*. When mechanical stress is placed on some area of the body, such as when the foot hits the ground in walking, a mechanical signal is sent to the bones where it is converted into an electrical signal. In turn, the mini-electric current literally draws calcium as well as other minerals into its bone, increasing both strength and density. When you decide to take the stairs to your office instead of the elevator, or carry groceries across the parking lot to your car, you are initiating the piezoelectric effect!

To prevent typical forms of osteoporosis, you need to exercise the long bones of the body—those of the thighs, calves, and upper and lower arms. Playing tennis, biking, and lifting a turkey out of the oven are all good ways to exercise these bones. The benefits of such exercise are site specific. To strengthen the leg bones, you must exercise your legs. However, swimming does not provide the same benefits as biking, because the body floats in water. Although doing laps is great aerobic exercise for the heart and lungs, the bones don't have to do the work of resisting gravity and consequently do not benefit in the same way.

Exercise is particularly effective if coupled with calcium supplements or hormone replacement therapy. In a controlled 2-year study, published in 1991 in the *New England Journal of Medicine*, researchers assessed the effects of exercise on 120 postmenopausal women, ages 52 to 60, with low bone density. Results of the study showed that a combination of exercise plus calcium slowed bone loss, while exercise coupled with supplemental hormones prevented bone loss. However, side effects such as breast tenderness and vaginal bleeding were more common among the women taking hormones.

Easy Does It

Use exercise to have a kind and friendly relationship with your body. Be sure not to use exercise as a reason to beat yourself up! You've probably been told, "no pain, no gain," but you will benefit much more in the long term if you exercise at your own pace.

- When you are doing aerobic exercise and breathing heavily, you should still be able to sing a little song to yourself. If you can't get the words out, you are pushing your body too much.

- If you are lifting weights, choose weights that are easy for you to lift and do more repetitions, rather than using weights that make you strain and that you can only lift two or three times. The amount of weight you hold in your hand puts many times the pressure on your shoulder joint. These tissues can be easily damaged, since this area of a woman's body is likely to be poorly developed. If you want to prove to yourself just how much you can lift, increase weights slowly and preferably under the supervision of a trainer.

- If you've just begun some sort of exercise routine, resist the temptation to be a star in your first session. When you feel tired or strained, cut back. You don't want to exhaust yourself so that you need to wait a week before exercising again, or risk injury. Choose a type of exercise that is appropriate for your capabilities and your interests.

Even Modest Levels of Physical Activity Are Beneficial

According to the American Heart Association, simply moving rather than not moving as you go about your day has a health-protective effect. Here are some good habits:

- At work, use the stairs rather than the elevator.
- Park your car at the far end of the parking lot when you go to the store to give yourself a little stroll.
- Pump your own gas.
- Park a few blocks from your destination and walk the rest of the way.
- When you receive a telephone call, stand to talk instead of sitting.
- If you are spending the evening on the couch watching television, during the commercials quickly do some household chore like putting away pots and pans, checking if doors are locked for the night, removing linens from the dryer and folding them, or exercising for a few minutes.
- Enjoy a walk after dinner.

A QUICK LOOK AT EXERCISES FOR MENOPAUSE

Hot Flashes

yoga

tai chi

qigong

aerobic exercise

Fatigue

yoga

aerobic exercise

qigong

Emotional Symptoms (anxiety, irritability, mood swings, depression)

yoga

tai chi

qigong

aerobic exercise

Poor Memory

yoga

aerobic exercise

Vaginal Changes and Lowered Sex Drive

yoga

aerobic exercise

Osteoporosis

yoga

tai chi

weight-bearing, low-impact aerobic exercise

As mentioned, exercise is a great way to reduce stress, which can worsen menopausal symptoms. The next chapter explores stress reduction in detail, the fifth step of the Healthy Menopause Program.

CHAPTER EIGHT

Step 5: Stress Management and Menopause

Stress can sometimes trigger symptoms of menopause and increase their severity. If you are approaching menopause, keep this connection in mind. As an article published in 1994 in *Experimental Gerontology* states, "Evidence that stress conditions have profound effect on reproductive function is suggestive that stress adaptation is important to understanding menopause problems." When you begin to have menopausal symptoms, evaluate if they are stress related.

Stress may be either physical or emotional. Physical stress can result from overexertion, heat, cold, and traumas such as surgery or an accident. Emotional stressors include pain, anxiety, excitement, and depression. A trying commute in traffic may make you especially irritable. An argument at work or the threat of a reprimand from your boss can bring on a hot flash. In a controlled laboratory setting, researchers observed that stress can trigger hot flashes, according to a study published in 1990 in *Health Psychology*. Scientists observed 21 postmenopausal women who reported having frequent hot flashes. When stressed, these women had significantly more hot flashes than during periods of nonstress.

A debate continues about which comes first, the symptom or the stress, and whether some problems blamed on menopause are actually due to stress alone. It is becoming clear that an inability to manage stress can color your experience of menopause. For this reason, the fifth step of the Healthy Menopause Program focuses on ways to better cope with everyday challenges and upset.

Your Adrenal Glands and Menopause

Any discussion of stress must begin with a description of the adrenals, two small glands, one above each kidney. If you reach behind you with each hand and touch your back a few inches above your waistline on either side of your backbone, you will be feeling the general area of your adrenals. Each gland consists of two separate portions: an inner medulla and an outer cortex.

The adrenal glands play a pivotal role in a wide array of body functions. They are involved in food digestion, especially sugars and starches, and they work in tandem with the thyroid gland, helping to generate and maintain energy levels. In terms of menopause, the ability of the adrenals to perform these tasks is very important. As explained in Chapter 5, faulty sugar metabolism can lead to and worsen menopausal symptoms. In addition, sluggish thyroid function, discussed in chapter 10, can make the transition of menopause more troublesome.

The adrenal glands produce 28 different hormones, including adrenaline, as part of the stress response. The primary raw material from which the adrenals produce these hormones, prior to menopause, is progesterone. During a woman's reproductive years, progesterone is in ample supply as the ovaries produce this hormone every time ovulation occurs. However, postmenopause, when a woman is no longer ovulating, progesterone levels fall. As a result, the adrenal glands come to rely more on another precursor hormone, androstenedione, made by the adrenals themselves.

Androstenedione travels to various locations: the fatty tissues of the belly, the liver, skeletal tissue, the kidneys, the brain, and hair follicles. At these various sites, especially in fatty tissues, this precursor hormone is converted to a form of estrogen, estrone. The quantity produced contributes significantly to a woman's hormone supply postmenopause, helping balance hormones and relieve menopausal symptoms. Thus, you have good reason to maintain healthy adrenal function and observe the recommendations for healthy lifestyle given in this chapter.

New research also suggests that stress hormones and sex hormones have an effect on each other. Animal studies show a close relationship between stress hormones and changes in estrogen levels. Estrogen affects the metabolism of the stress hormone norepinephrine, which is also produced in the brain, as well as the neurotransmitter serotonin. These are functionally important in areas of the hypothalamus that regulate body temperature, patterns of sleep, and mood. Estrogen also affects the metabolism of endorphins, compounds that generate a feeling of well-being. One theory of hot flashes is that lower levels of estrogen lead to lower levels of these natural opiates, which in turn stimulate hot flashes. How this occurs is currently being investigated. There may also be an association between estrogen levels and levels of catecholestrogens, recently discovered compounds that potentially influence mood. This association may be one of the origins of mood and sleep disturbances that occur with menopause.

Having Some Stress Is Essential for Health

A healthy level of stress is a stimulant that keeps your system functioning. Stress keeps you energized, sharp-witted, and physically active, which in turn supports health. As your body goes into alert, blood pressure and heart rate increase. The metabolism of protein, fats, and carbohydrates increases to provide ready energy. In contrast, a lack of stress can be debilitating. It is well known that when patients remain confined to bed for weeks and even months at a time, physical strength is lost, bones weaken, and even thinking processes can slow.

However, in our modern society, few people suffer from too little stress! Most people have become accustomed to a level of challenge and excitement in their daily lives and in the type of leisure activities they choose that promotes stress overload. While having some stress supports health, too much undermines well-being. Where the dividing line falls between enough and too much was first delineated by the great Dr. Hans Selye, the pioneering endocrinologist who defined the very concept of stress in the 1930s.

The Three Stages of Stress

According to Selye, in the first stage of stress the body prepares for fight or flight. This alarm reaction kept our distant ancestors alert and helped enable them to survive a multitude of physical dangers ranging from treacherous terrain to night predators. The adrenals pump out extra amounts of hormones, triggering the release of blood glucose to provide extra energy for the emergency situation. Then, when the crisis is over, the adrenals once again quiet down and the body has a chance to rest and repair.

However, after being exposed to stress for a long period of time, the body goes into the second stage, which is the resistance stage of stress. The adrenals adapt to prolonged stress by increasing in size, thereby enhancing function. At the same time, the adrenals require a greater amount of nutrients to perform their many functions and body reserves must be drawn upon. Eventually, the body can run low on both nutrients and energy. This resistance stage of stress can last for weeks, months, and even years.

The third stage of stress is adrenal exhaustion. Adrenal function slows until the natural antistress responses of the body kick in slowly if at all. Reserves of both nutrients and energy are used up. Our society is full of people who are running on empty because of adrenal exhaustion. Unhealthy substances that can help an individual sustain such over-the-top living are readily available—caffeine, sugar, colas, and nicotine.

Midlife Stress

Although according to research, life is not necessarily more stressful at midlife than at any other period, most women would agree that it is a challenging time. For starters, menopause itself can be a source of stress. The purely physical changes that occur with menopause can draw on reserves. When a woman is younger, the body produces sufficient progesterone to help replenish adrenal hormones. But postmenopause, this reserve is greatly diminished, potentially making women much less tolerant of stress. Entering menopause in a state of adrenal exhaustion, a woman can be caught in a downward cycle of progesterone deficiency, resulting in estrogen dominance and related symptoms, as well as exhaustion. Characteristic signs of this depletion are weakness, fatigue, irritability, and mental sluggishness.

In addition, night sweats that significantly disrupt sleep can result in some of the more serious psychological problems associated with menopause. Women who seem to go "crazy" during menopause may simply be suffering from sleep deprivation. Males are also susceptible to lack of sleep. In one study, men were awakened each time they fell into deep REM (rapid eye movement) sleep, the phase during which dreaming takes place. To feel refreshed and rested, REM sleep is essential. After 3 days of being deprived of this restorative form of sleep, the men showed distinct signs of psychosis.

Midlife often brings stressful changes other than menopause. For women who gave birth around age 30, children are now grown and begin to leave home. The empty nest syndrome can take its toll. Sometimes couples at midlife reassess their marriages and decide to divorce. Or a woman may begin to lose interest in her work.

What menopause means to you can also be a source of stress. Women in Western societies are often saddled with negative attitudes toward menopause. Centuries ago, in Europe, it was thought that evil humors such as melancholy remained in women at menopause, turning them into witches. Today, menopause is linked to growing old in many women's minds. And although Norma Desmond, in the movie *Sunset Boulevard*, is an extreme example of the demise of the aging woman, the ghost of Norma Desmond still haunts many women in our youth-oriented culture.

Using Diet and Nutrients to Help Manage Stress

Key to managing stress at menopause is nutrition. Although few studies to date address the relationship between stress, menopause, and diet, much is known about the health of the adrenal glands and diet. Chapter 5 goes into detail about the foods to eat to support adrenal function. But briefly, nutrients that are essential for adrenal function include vitamin A, B complex, and vitamin C. And you'll find in the average supermarket a wealth of foods that supply these, including sweet potatoes, mushrooms, avocado, lobster, and chicken.

Foods That Stress the Adrenals

In addition to choosing foods that help the body handle stress, it's important to avoid foods that undermine adrenal function. For instance, refined sugar and refined flour deplete some nutrients that are vital for adrenal function. Caffeine also depletes the system of vitamins and minerals, and overstimulates the adrenal glands. Unfortunately, some of these foods show up in virtually every meal.

To be converted to energy, refined sugar requires thiamin, riboflavin, niacin, and pantothenic acid. But refined white sugar provides none of these, consequently depleting body reserves. High consumption of sugar can burden the adrenals by competing for available vitamins and robbing the adrenals of the supply they need for proper functioning. Corn syrup and the many other refined sweeteners used in thousands of food products also lack B vitamins. Given the amount of sugar North Americans eat, the effect of this intake on adrenal function is significant.

When flour is refined, approximately 22 nutrients are partially removed and only 6 or 7 are returned to "enrich" it—and not necessarily as much as the original grain contained. Compared with refined flour, whole wheat and brown rice have higher amounts of B vitamins, which support adrenal function and help you physically manage stress.

Caffeine has a stimulating effect on organs and tissues within a few minutes of being consumed. The caffeine in a beverage acts directly on individual cells, affecting the chemical reactions within them. For instance, in the adrenals, caffeine triggers the synthesis and release of the two stress hormones, epinephrine and norepinephrine, stimulating a classic stress response. These hormones cause sugars stored in the cells to be released into the bloodstream and metabolized to produce energy—the rush of energy that caffeine typically provides. Caffeinated coffee and tea are also diuretics, triggering the loss of the water-soluble vitamins, beta-carotene, the B vitamins, and vitamin C via the urine. A woman feeling the effects of too much caffeine is likely to have symptoms that are also associated with menopause—anxiety, irritability, and restlessness.

Chamomile: The Herb for Stress

You can always rely on this gentle herb to be relaxing. It takes about 5 minutes to boil the water and brew the tea and can put you at ease for hours. Carry some chamomile tea bags in your purse. When you eat out, order a cup of hot water and make your own tea rather than ordering coffee.

When preparing herbal tea, be aware that tea made in the usual fashion, with one tea bag per cup, is actually quite weak. For a stronger, more effective infusion, use 2 or 3 tea bags per cup of water and steep them at least five minutes.

Relaxation First-Aid Kit

Be prepared for those times when stress overtakes you. Ready your bathing area for an emergency bubble bath. Keep a list of places you love to go and give yourself a treat for a few hours when you feel overwhelmed. Line up a good massage therapist to knead your troubles away. And be ready to do some deep breathing, a proven relaxation technique you can practice anytime, anywhere.

Meditation

Many people use yoga as a preparation for meditation. When the postures are completed, the mind and body are ready for some quiet time. Meditation is the practice of being in the moment and silencing the chatter of the brain. Switching off the usual mind-talk this way has been shown to reduce stress. Studies conducted by physiologist R. Keith Wallace have proven that meditation can have profound effects not only on reducing stress but also on reversing the aging process itself.

Inventing a New You

In the North American culture, the role of both the maiden and the mother are honored. These archetypes embody youthfulness, beauty, and sexuality. But after menopause, where do you go with your life? When you think of aging and being postmenopausal, what images come to mind? Do you conjure up pictures of witches you once saw in illustrated children's books? Or do you first think of those over-the-hill women, the "before" shots that advertisers like to feature in ads selling wrinkle creams and drugs to prevent osteoporosis? You don't have to buy into these stereotypes.

Come up with your own positive images of what you'll be like after menopause. Bestow on yourself the dignity and tender care you deserve. Have some fun with this process:

- Make a collage using images of women you admire, things you love such as mountains and flowers, words that evoke qualities you would like to have. Keep this collage on your wall and live with these pictures while they sink into your mind. They are your goals.

- Make a list of how you don't want your life to be as you age. Then write a list of the opposite statements and make these your goals. ("I'll be fat and my joints will be stiff" becomes "I'll have a healthy weight and be able to move and stretch freely.")

- Talk with friends and come up with some new ideas about aging that you can support each other in achieving.

When you begin to let your mind wander over the dire consequences of menopause, take this as a cue! Substitute positive images for outdated ones. Stepping into this new phase of your life, standing tall, shoulders squared, can make menopause all that much easier.

Write your own script and let the story of Valerie be an inspiration. At midlife, Valerie found herself back at home, living with her aging mother who recently had had a stroke. For Valerie, the stress of suddenly being a caretaker, coupled with the onset of menopause, was overwhelming. She also began to feel housebound, as family funds ran out and her mother could no longer afford a nurse, keeping Valerie at home most days. Valerie investigated her local neighborhood and found a charming dance studio nearby. She was amazed that just 1 hour spent moving to music could dispel her worries and cares so quickly. Valerie talked about this with the other women in her class and found to her surprise that the other women were also using the exercise class more as a form of stress management than as a way to get in shape! Being very creative, Valerie took this concept one step further and began to take Hawaiian dancing lessons, a fantasy since her teenage years. She became quite good at this and began to hire out as an entertainer at parties, also putting time into concocting tropical costumes. Valerie appreciated the humor in such a turn of events and brought her exuberance for dancing, music, and color into her mother's life as well. What began as a desperate attempt to break out of a limited situation ended up transforming her life.

CHAPTER NINE

Step 6: Hormone Replacement Therapy

For many women, the treatment of choice for menopause symptoms and the prevention of diseases of aging is hormone replacement therapy (HRT). Most likely, if you discuss menopause with your physician, you will be offered some form of supplemental hormones. However, while many benefits of taking hormone replacement therapy are well known, questions remain about its long-term safety and side effects. As future research provides more information about the pros and cons of taking hormones, physicians may be able to recommend HRT with more certainty. But no matter how much evidence or research a doctor gathers, each woman ultimately must make this vitally important decision for herself, either by discussing the option of hormones with an open-minded physician, or, if given a prescription, deciding on her own whether to fill it!

This chapter tells you about the various forms of hormone

treatment available. It explores the benefits and side effects of these and updates you on current research.

The Beginnings of
Hormone Replacement Therapy

In 1938, an inexpensive form of estrogen was distilled from plant sources. Prescribed to treat menopause, the hormone could be taken orally and did not require an injection. However, it was not until the 1950s and early 1960s that Robert Wilson, a physician, popularized the use of estrogen replacement therapy (ERT). With seemingly unlimited enthusiasm, he was in favor of prescribing estrogen well before menopause began so that a woman would never experience symptoms of the change. He even recommended estrogen for such conditions as acne and "sexual underdevelopment," and often prescribed very large dosages.

Then in the mid-1970s, case histories began to appear in medical journals showing an association between taking estrogen alone, without progesterone, and an increased risk of developing endometrial cancer. These observations spurred researchers to find a safer way to administer estrogen. Eventually, they discovered that taking progesterone along with estrogen could significantly eliminate this cancer risk. By the end of the decade, hormone replacement therapy was once again given the green light.

Today, the most commonly prescribed estrogen, Premarin, is a conjugated equine estrogen derived from the urine of pregnant mares. Many women find this method of production an insurmountable obstacle to taking the drug because of the possible mistreatment of the animals. There are also synthetic and semisynthetic estrogen compounds available, including Ogen and Estrace. (For more information on supplemental estrogen, see page 159.)

Benefits of Estrogen and Progesterone

Supplemental hormones offer many benefits, substantiated by a growing body of research. Hormone replacement therapy impacts the reproductive system and can ease and even eliminate symptoms of menopause.

Estrogen

Estrogen can dramatically reduce the frequency and severity of hot flashes after a few weeks of supplementation. ERT also helps a woman avoid the fatigue that may result from persistent hot flashes, as well as night sweats. Moods even out. And supplemental estrogen counteracts the thinning and dryness of vaginal tissue, which can make intercourse uncomfortable. The vagina once again becomes lubricated. A woman's outer skin also becomes more moist and better retains elasticity.

Studies show that supplemental estrogen helps restore verbal memory. Initial studies recently completed also indicate that estrogen can lower the risk of developing Alzheimer's and other forms of dementia.

Urinary tract infections tend to increase after menopause due to tissue changes. Burning and irritation during urination is more likely. Estrogen can reverse these symptoms. However, there is no proof that estrogen alleviates urinary incontinence, which is common postmenopause. This problem is more related to age than hormone deficiency.

Using supplemental estrogen is also one way to reduce the risk of osteoporosis and, in some cases, heart disease. (More information about this is given later in the chapter.)

Progesterone

Progesterone can be useful in reducing hot flashes and in certain circumstances is the preferred hormone of choice. During perimenopause, when a woman can begin to experience her first hot flashes, her estrogen levels may be relatively high and taking more estrogen would only create more hormone imbalance.

Supplementing with progesterone can also prevent excessive menstrual bleeding (menorrhagia), which can sometimes occur during perimenopause if a woman has become anovulatory (no longer producing eggs), or has a defective luteal phase of her menstrual cycle (when progesterone is normally produced). However, also be aware that menorrhagia may not be related to progesterone levels. Heavy bleeding can occur for a variety of other reasons, including stress, obesity, uterine fibroids, and hypothryroidism.

Using Hormone Replacement Therapy

Both estrogen and progesterone come in a variety of forms. Working with your physician, you can experiment with these to find what works best for you. Here's what you have to choose from.

Supplementing with Estrogen

You have your choice of synthetic estrogens and natural estrogens. There is frequently some confusion about what these two terms mean. For the record, both types of estrogen are synthesized in laboratories. Most synthetic estrogens are made from the urine of pregnant mares. They have a molecular structure that slightly differs from your body's own estrogen; thus, pharmaceutical companies can patent these compounds. Natural estrogens, in contrast, have the same chemical configuration as the estrogen women normally produce—that is, estradiol, estrone, and estriol.

Types of Supplemental Estrogen and Their Routes of Delivery

You can take estrogen in a variety of forms, whether you are taking estrogen alone or a combination of estrogen and progesterone. The pill form is the most common, followed by the patch and vaginal cream. Estrogens are also available in gels, as sublinguals, and as injectable pellets. Premarin, which comes in pill form, is the most frequently prescribed estrogen. This preparation consists mainly of mixed estrogens derived from a pregnant mare's urine; hence the trade name. Some of the hormones, such as *equilin*, are not naturally present in humans, but once ingested, the body converts these to estradiol.

Premarin was first introduced in 1941 and has been used in the great majority of experiments focusing on supplemental hormones.

PILLS

All drugs taken orally, including estradiol in pill form, move from the intestines and travel immediately to the liver in high concentration, before continuing on to other areas of the body. In the case of estradiol, the liver breaks down some of the estradiol to estrone and other forms of estrogen.

There can be problems with this route of delivery. Estrogen, once ingested, can accumulate in the digestive tract. Here it can be chemically transformed by bacteria, which can change the type and potency of the estrogen the body eventually receives. This route of delivery requires that the liver be optimally functioning, which may not be the case. Liver function may not be up to par if a woman's diet is high in sugar, fat, or alcohol, and is lacking in the B-complex vitamins. In addition, the pill form of estradiol may not be appropriate if a woman has a history of liver disease, gallbladder disease, clotting problems, or hypertension.

The most common form of estrogen, estradiol, can also stimulate the liver to produce large quantities of potentially harmful substances, such as cholesterol, and proteins that promote clotting. Because of these problems, purified estrone is sometimes prescribed instead. Estrone pills consist of the compound estropipate, which is available in a generic form, Ortho-Est tablets, and is sold under the trade name Ogen. This product has less of an effect on the liver's production of proteins than other oral estrogens.

Premarin is a conjugated estrogen, that is, a mix of types of estrogen. When you take Premarin, you have the benefit of taking an extensively studied medication for which the benefits and side effects are well known. Premarin is also available in a wider range of dosages than any other estrogen product, allowing a physician more options in tailoring a prescription to your needs. Another option is Estratab, an esterified estrone type of estrogen synthesized from soy and wild yam. Estratab has the same potency and uses, and is available in the same dosages as Premarin. Esterified estrogens break down more slowly in the bloodstream thereby providing a steadier supply of hormones.

The usual recommended dosage for estrogen is 0.625 milligrams; however, there are exceptions. For relief of symptoms, some women need as much as 0.9 to 1.25 milligrams of estrogen. Other women, to avoid side effects, need to cut their dosage to as low as 0.3 milligrams.

In the standard protocol, oral estrogen is taken for 25 days each month, followed by a week of no estrogen, before this cycle is repeated. Unfortunately, the break in treatment can bring on menopausal symptoms such as hot flashes. Another oral estrogen protocol is to take the pill continuously without a week off. Taking estrogen without progesterone can increase a woman's risk of uterine cancer and is only recommended if your uterus has been removed.

THE PATCH

An alternative to the pill is the patch, a small, round piece of adhesive several inches wide. Each patch holds estrogen that passes across a membrane and is absorbed transdermally (through the skin) and into the bloodstream. (The skin is the largest organ of elimination in the body and is also a ready avenue of absorption.)

The advantage of the patch over the pill is that the estrogen it delivers is absorbed directly into the general circulation, rather than first traveling to the liver. Lower dosages can be prescribed and the patch also delivers a steadier flow of hormones than the pill, more closely mimicking the body's own production of estrogen. Consequently transdermal estrogen is less likely to trigger menopausal symptoms. In addition, this form of estrogen offers some protection against osteoporosis and heart disease, although the latter benefit is now controversial.

Transdermal estrogen is marketed under the names Estraderm and Climara, which contain estradiol. It is a good choice for women who have had a history of gallbladder or liver disease, as well as problems with high blood pressure and blood clotting, unless clotting factors are abnormal.

The patch is available in a range of dosages from 0.0375 to 0.1 milligram. The patch is applied directly to the skin on certain key areas of the body that readily absorb the hormone— the abdomen, the thighs, and the buttocks. The patch must be changed twice a week, and with each application the patch must be placed in a new location. It can cause skin irritation, but rotating its placement can help prevent this.

As with the pill, the patch needs to be used in conjunction with progesterone to reduce the risk of uterine cancer.

ESTROGEN VAGINAL CREAM

Estrogen vaginal cream is applied to the vagina and the urethral area, and is thereby absorbed into the bloodstream. Like the patch, this method of delivery also avoids the intestinal tract and the liver, and eliminates related side effects. While estrogen vaginal cream can affect various parts of the body, it is primarily used to reduce thinning of the vaginal walls and to restore these tissues to a healthier and more youthful condition. The cream can increase vaginal lubrication, making sexual activity more comfortable.

However, a drawback of vaginal cream is that its effects are not as predictable as other forms of supplemental estrogen. Estrogens can be absorbed into the system in widely varying amounts, determined by the thickness of the vaginal wall. The effect of vaginal cream is also not sufficient to significantly reduce the risk of heart disease or osteoporosis. Using a cream can be messy and the cream may soil clothing.

You also have the choice of using a natural estrogen cream, which can be used vaginally, as well as applied to various areas of the body. The estrogen is massaged into the thin, soft skin of the chest, stomach, inner arms and thighs, and neck. This cream is made from soybeans that contain estrogenic compounds. Natural estrogen cream contains sitosterol, a form of estrone. It offers the advantages of any natural hormone product, and like any transdermal product, it is effective at lower doses.

One of the most common estrogen vaginal cream products is Premarin cream. It is applied using an applicator that can deliver 1.25 to 2.5 milligrams of estrogen to the tissues of the vagina; however, smaller doses are often sufficient. Some women find that they benefit most by using estrogen cream every day for a week or two until their vaginal tissue begins to respond. At this point, using the cream only twice or three times a week is usually sufficient. Estropipate, which metabolizes to estrone, is also available as a cream.

If you decide to use natural estrogen cream, the starting dosage is ¼ teaspoon a day, which supplies approximately 1.85 milligrams of estrogen. This dosage can be slowly increased until symptoms abate. You can then reduce the dosage to the minimum needed to prevent symptoms.

As with the other forms of supplemental estrogen, you also need to take progesterone to prevent cancer of the uterus. Supplementing with progesterone, at least every 3 months, can help achieve a balance of hormones and prevent the lining of the uterus from thickening or becoming precancerous.

SPECIALTY PHARMACIES

Specialty pharmacies are a source of natural hormones. Such companies hand-compound estradiol and estrone in dosages not commonly available. Specialty pharmacies also prepare customized combinations of these hormones (see Resources for a list of compounding pharmacies).

Compounding pharmacies are also a source of estriol, another natural hormone. Estriol is less potent than the other two types of estrogen; therefore, estriol is given in higher doses. It is considered the safest estrogen in terms of breast cancer. Based on population studies, women who live in countries with a low rate of breast cancer tend to have higher levels of estriol. Estriol has even been used successfully to reverse the progress of advanced breast cancer. Although research to date is limited, estriol appears to be an attractive option to other estrogens on the market. It is also the major estrogen in Dr. Jonathan Wright's "Tri-Est," an estrogen replacement formula for postmenopausal women.

Available through compounding pharmacies (see Resources), Tri-Est is 80% estriol, 10% estradiol, and 10% estrone, supplying the three forms of estrogen the body produces and in the same proportions. These natural estrogens are weaker than Premarin, so a dosage four times the strength of Premarin is required. Application as a cream is most effective.

In general, natural estrogens appear to provide the same benefits as Premarin, lessening hot flashes, and lowering the risk of osteoporosis and, in some cases, heart disease. However, relatively few studies have been conducted to test natural estrogens, compared with Premarin, and more information needs to be gathered on their side effects and bioavailability.

Side Effects of Estrogen Replacement Therapy

Estrogen has an impact on many body systems besides reproductive function. Estrogen receptors have been identified in the liver, in bones, nerves, vascular smooth muscle cells, and heart cells, indicating its multiple functions and perhaps providing a partial explanation for why taking hormones can result in such a variety of side effects. These range from mild problems such as increased fatigue to various potentially life-threatening diseases. Possible side effects include:

- Changes in the pattern of menstrual bleeding
- Breakthrough bleeding and spotting
- Fluid retention and weight gain
- Breast tenderness and enlargement
- Anxiety
- Changes in sex drive

Supplementing with estrogen can increase the risk of certain diseases and conditions, such as:

- Endometrial cancer
- Breast cancer
- Tendency to develop blood clots
- Lupus erythematosus
- Ovarian cancer
- Gallbladder disease

In some women, estrogen can promote an increased suscep-tibility to vaginal yeast infection, fibrocystic breast disease, increased blood pressure, decreased tolerance of blood sugar, skin rash, headaches, migraines, and dizziness. Nausea, vomiting, and abdominal cramps may also occur. There may be changes in the cornea of the eye, making it difficult to wear contact lenses. A woman may experience an increased sensitivity to sunlight and be more sensitive to synthetics and additives.

Estrogen may also not be appropriate if a woman has a large fibroid tumor in her uterus, a common problem in women after age 40. Elevated levels of estrogen promote fibroid growth.

Supplementing with Progesterone

Progesterone plays an important part in the reproductive cycle. When ovulation occurs, the ovaries produce copious amounts of progesterone, which helps to prepare the uterus to receive a fertilized egg. If fertilization occurs, progesterone levels remain high and the placenta becomes a primary source of progesterone. A very small amount of progesterone is also produced by the adrenal glands.

But not all progesterones are the same, and you need to be aware of the differences. Pharmaceutical companies sell a synthetic hormone, progestin, which like synthetic estrogen, has a chemical structure that differs somewhat from your body's own progesterone. You may also sometimes see the terms *progestagen*, and *progestogen*, which are also both synthetic. The first progestins were compounded in the 1950s, but were initially contaminated with a form of estrogen. Eventually, purer progestins became available. The change in structure allows the drug companies to patent these products. You need to be aware that this synthetic progestin is commonly referred to as *progesterone*, which strictly speaking it is not.

Synthetic progestins can cause problems. Most of the

unpleasant side effects women experience from HRT are from progestins, not estrogens. They can actually worsen menopausal symptoms such as fatigue, fluid retention, breast tenderness, and depression. Synthetic progestins can also raise cholesterol.

Types of Synthetic Progesterone

Progestins are classified into two groups: the 19-nor-testosterone derivatives; and the C-21 progestins, dydrogesterone and medroxyprogesterone acetate. In 1951, the first 19-nortestosterone compound, norethindrone, was extracted from androgens. Generic names for these are norgestrel and levonorgestrel, sold under the trade names Aygestin, Norlutate, Norlutin, Ovrett, and Micronor.

Medroxyprogesterone acetate was first developed as a contraceptive, Depo-Provera, and has been available since the late 1960s. The best-known form of medroxyprogesterone is Provera. Other brand names are Amen and Curretab.

The most common regimen is to add progestins to the last 10 to 14 days of each cycle. However, this can result in side effects including nausea, breast tenderness, headaches, and breakthrough bleeding.

The minimal dosage is 5 to 10 milligrams a day, to prevent the proliferation of cells in the lining of the uterus. If this amount produces fatigue and depression, the dosage may need to be reduced to as low as 1.25 milligrams a day.

Compared with the progesterone your body makes, synthetic progestins can be 10 to 100 times more potent! These products may also have some estrogenic effects.

Supplementing with Natural Progesterone and Routes of Delivery

Natural progesterone has the exact same chemical configuration as the progesterone produced by a woman's body. Be sure to take natural progesterone in a micronized form because unaltered natural progesterone is destroyed by stomach acids. Only micronized progesterone can be absorbed and used by the body. Micronized natural progesterone is widely used in Europe and is becoming more popular in North America. This form of progesterone seems to be as effective at protecting against endometrial cancer as synthetic progesterone. It seems to have a gentler effect on the system and does not cause as many side effects as progestins. However, drowsiness can result as natural progesterone can act as a sedative. In addition, in women who are especially sensitive, it may cause dizziness.

Natural progesterone is usually produced using extracts of phytohormones found in abundant amounts in soybeans or Mexican wild yams. (Because a manufacturing process is involved, this form of progesterone is sometimes categorized as being semisynthetic.)

In England, natural progesterone alone has been used for decades to treat PMS. In the United States, in one small study, oral capsules of micronized progesterone were shown to ease symptoms of menopause while causing minimal side effects. And in a large study, the PEPI Study, in 1995, this form of progesterone, compared with progestins, was found to be more effective at lowering blood fats, a risk factor for heart disease. Natural progesterone, which is pharmaceutical grade, comes in many forms including micronized pills, creams, gels, suppositories, injectables, and pellets.

Natural progesterone can be taken as an oral capsule with an oil base, wax suppositories, a rectal fluid inserted via syringe, sublingual lozenges or capsules, by injection, and even as a nasal spray.

A typical dosage of micronized natural progesterone is 200 to 300 milligrams a day, given in a divided dose. It is normally taken for 10 to 14 days each month. Natural progesterone is also available as a vaginal or rectal suppository, with 25 to 50 milligrams taken twice daily, and as an over-the-counter cream. The cream is absorbed transdermally and is stored in fat cells. The progesterone is then gradually released from these reservoirs and travels through the blood to progesterone receptor sites.

A popular brand is Progest, which is taken in a usual dosage of ¼ to ½ teaspoon in the morning and at night. The cream is applied to the body where the skin is soft and thin, such as the abdomen, breasts, inner arms and thighs, wrist, face, and nape of the neck. If you find that the cream is absorbed in under 2 minutes, you may need to use more.

The stronger natural progesterone preparations, such as micronized progesterone pills, can be up to 30 times more potent than some creams that contain progesterone precursors from plants. The stronger preparations tend to be available only by prescription.

In addition, some over-the-counter products only contain progesterone precursors from plant sources. Manufacturers may claim that these products are a reliable source of pro-gesterone because intestinal bacteria convert these compounds into progesterone. However, many experts deny this conversion ever takes place. Products that contain only plant precursors of progesterone are equivalent to taking an herbal preparation and provide the weakest effects on the system.

To differentiate between these products and those that contain the active hormone, the Food and Drug Administration (FDA) now requires a manufacturer to include the word *progesterone* on the label when the hormone itself is actually in the product. Check labels when you shop.

Side Effects of Supplementing with Progesterone

Taking progesterone can lead to many of the same side effects as taking estrogen. Synthetic progestins can promote PMS-like symptoms such as anxiety and depression, as well as bloating. In some cases, fatigue, headaches, and dizziness may also occur. Related medical conditions can include allergic rash, jaundice (a sign of liver toxicity), stroke, and blood clots in the legs and lungs. Progestins can also decrease the absorption of nutrients such as vitamin B_6, which plays an important role in the health of the reproductive system. Natural progesterone also has potential side effects: breast tenderness, sedation, dizziness and light-headedness, pimples, and increased sensitivity of the eyes.

Combining Estrogen with Progesterone

If you are taking estrogen and you have a uterus that is intact, you also need to supplement with progesterone to avoid an increased risk of uterine cancer. Estrogen stimulates the growth of the endometrial cells that line the uterus. An accelerated rate of growth results in the buildup of the endometrial layer. Normally this process is counteracted by the sloughing off of tissues that is triggered by progesterone. An endometrial layer that is thick and growing is more likely to become cancerous if progesterone is not present to cause these cells to shed. (Also read the section on breast cancer later in this chapter for information about the possible effects of progesterone on other types of cancer.)

- Many health professionals recommend using both estrogen and progesterone in a pattern that mimics the menstrual cycle. Use estrogen from day 1 to day 25 and progesterone from day 10 to day 25. Then take no hormones for the next 5 to 7 days. On this protocol, women who have not undergone a hysterectomy continue to menstruate or again begin to menstruate, because the progesterone triggers the shedding of the uterine lining. There will be some evidence of withdrawal bleeding for months, or years depending on factors such as age, hormonal status, weight, and family history. However, eventually, menstruation will gradually taper off to minimal or stop completely.

- An equally common protocol is to take estrogen on a daily basis along with small amounts of progestins. This scheduling does not bring on menstruation. However, a woman may experience breakthrough bleeding if hormone levels are not balanced. One shortcoming of continuous supplementation is that no studies exist documenting the long-term effects of taking hormones this way.

- Another routine is to take estrogen for the first half of the month, from day 1 to day 14, and then progesterone from day 14 to day 18. This scheduling of hormones is associated with withdrawal bleeding.

Testosterone: The "Male" Hormone for Women

While testosterone is the primary male sex hormone, associated with sexual drive and aggressive behavior, women also produce some testosterone. The ovaries are the primary source of testosterone in women prior to menopause and continue to produce this hormone postmenopause, although in dwindling amounts.

As in men, testosterone in women increases libido. In addition, this hormone stimulates a healthy appetite, strengthens muscles, and generally promotes well-being. Physicians will sometimes prescribe testosterone along with estrogen for women who have lost their sex drive following natural menopause or a hysterectomy.

However, testosterone can have unwelcome side effects. If taken over a long period of time, these hormones can be masculinizing. Body and facial hair may increase and high doses may lead to enlargement of the clitoris, deepening of the voice, and an increase in muscle mass—changes that may be irreversible even when the supplements are stopped.

Testosterone, in the form of synthetic androgen methy-testosterone, can be taken orally as a capsule. Each capsule contains 10 milligrams of hormone. Therapy is usually started at 10 milligrams a day and is gradually increased to a limit of 50 milligrams a day. The downside of orally administered testosterone is that it is poorly absorbed in the digestive tract.

Natural testosterone is prepared as a cream and as a gel, the two most popular forms. The cream is applied to the skin, and once absorbed, enters the general circulation and travels directly to target cells, helping to ensure its potency. Only later does the testosterone pass through the liver, which breaks it down. Gels, usually applied to vaginal tissue, also enter the bloodstream directly.

Taking Hormones to Prevent Disease

Even if a woman's menopausal symptoms are not particularly troubling, physicians still recommend HRT to prevent and treat osteoporosis and heart disease. You need to assess these benefits when deciding about taking hormones. Of course, following a good diet, having sufficient exercise, and managing stress are all vitally important for your long-term health, but you may also want to consider adding hormones to your self-help program.

Osteoporosis

Bone loss, which begins to occur in a woman's 30s, accelerates at menopause, as estrogen levels abruptly decline. Osteoporosis can be particularly severe in women if they have surgery to remove the ovaries, a major source of estrogen. If a young woman undergoes hysterectomy that includes removal of the ovaries, weakening of bones can begin much earlier. (Chapter 10 more fully explains how this disease can develop and tells about lifestyle changes that can do much to ensure bone strength.)

Besides making dietary and lifestyle changes to prevent osteoporosis, some women add hormones to their regimen. Supplemental estrogen has been found to slow bone loss. But, to be beneficial, taking estrogen must be coupled with weight-bearing exercise such as riding a bicycle or walking. Taking in sufficient calcium is also important. (Suggested dosages are given in Chapter 4 on nutrients for menopause.)

Progesterone can even increase bone density. In a small study that tested the effects of natural progesterone on bone density, remarkable results were achieved, but the women in the study also supported their health through diet, nutritional supplements, and exercise.

The use of estrogen and progesterone together may be particularly beneficial. Bone loss may be completely prevented using this regimen. Benefits are greatest if treatment begins in the early stages of menopause, and, at minimum, starting within 3 years of when menopause begins. During the first years after menopause, bone loss is greatest.

Supplementation protects bones for as long as hormones are taken. However, as soon as a woman stops supplementing, bone loss resumes, possibly at accelerated rates. Women at high risk for osteoporosis may decide to stay on hormones throughout their life postmenopause. However, the drawback of this strategy is that continued use of estrogen may well be associated with a greater risk of breast cancer.

Heart Disease

Estrogen is routinely recommended to *prevent* cardiovascular disease, however, studies focusing on this association have yielded conflicting results. Research suggests that not all women need to follow this course, and that HRT may not be as protective as is commonly assumed.

Healthy women, without heart disease, have been the focus of much research. Over 30 studies, conducted since 1980, have shown that in these women, HRT/ERT lowers the risk of coronary disease by 20 to 50%. Hormones have improved blood levels of cholesterol and triglycerides, both heart disease risk factors. In the 1995 Postmenopausal Estrogen/Progestin Interventions (PEPI) Trial, hormones had a beneficial effect on lipid levels, blood pressure, and blood clotting. Such results led to the blanket recommendation that all postmenopausal women be placed on HRT/ERT to prevent cardiovascular disease.

Critics of this research pointed out the dangers of relying on changes in risk factors to prove the benefits of a treatment. They also argued that the women on estrogen were healthier to start and led a lifestyle known to prevent heart disease. A study published in 1996 in the *American Journal of Epidemiology* makes this case. The Heart and Estrogen-Progestin Replacement Study (HERS), the first large-scale, randomized, prospective trial on HRT/ERT and cardiovascular disease, further added to the uncertainty.

The HERS trial included 2763 older postmenopausal women with existing coronary artery disease (CAD). Hormones improved cholesterol levels. However, the decrease in CAD was not as great as would be predicted from the changes in cholesterol, challenging the notion that hormones prevent disease by improving such risk factors, and thereby putting the usefulness of other studies in doubt.

Further, during the first year of the study, the women taking hormones surprisingly had a higher death rate due to blood clots than those not on hormones. Replacement therapy was protective only after 4 or 5 years. Consequently, the American

Heart Association published a new guideline and warned against starting postmenopausal women with heart disease on estrogen. However, women with heart disease who have taken HRT/ERT for more than one year still have the green light for continuing use.

Certainly, more research is needed to determine the precise role of hormone levels postmenopause and the risk of heart disease. Fortunately, science has found solid evidence of the role that diet, exercise, and stress management play in heart healthy ways of preventing heart disease, which are discussed in other chapters.

The Link Between Supplemental Hormones and Breast Cancer

The risk of breast cancer has doubled since 1940. Today, a woman has a 1-in-9 *lifetime* chance of developing breast cancer. This does not mean that a woman, whatever her age, has this level of risk. Rather, the incidence of breast cancer is higher in older women who are part of a declining population. By age 85, the risk is 1-in-9, but a woman 50 years old has a risk of 1-in-50. By age 60, the risk is 1-in-23; by age 70, 1-in-13; and by age 80, 1-in-10.

Research suggests that estrogen replacement therapy does not increase the risk of breast cancer if supplementation continues for only a few years. But if estrogen is taken for 10 to 15 years, then a woman's risk of breast cancer increases 20 to 30%. Unfortunately, women using estrogen to prevent osteoporosis are told to continue taking estrogen into old age.

In addition, a recent and large study, published in 2000 in the *Journal of the American Medical Association*, found that a combined estrogen-progestin regimen increased the risk of breast cancer even more than estrogen alone. This study included 46,355 postmenopausal women who had participated in an earlier study conducted between 1973 and 1980. In the earlier study, the average age of the women was 58. Researchers conducted a follow-up assessment in 29 screening centers throughout the United States. While more studies are called for, these results are impressive and call into question taking progesterone along with estrogen, a regimen routinely recommended to avoid cancer of the uterus.

Of course, taking hormones is not the only risk factor for breast cancer. Other risk factors include early onset of menstruation, a late menopause, never becoming pregnant, and having family members with breast cancer. A high-fat diet and intake of more than 1 ounce of alcohol per day are also risk factors. Some experts believe that pesticides in food and in the environment promote breast cancer. These compounds can have powerful estrogenic effects once they enter the system. Eating organic foods is important to your health (see Chapter 5).

Supplemental Hormones and Drug Interactions

If you are on medication and are also taking hormones, drug interactions are possible. Check with your physician if you are taking estrogen along with anticoagulants or corticosteroids. Alcohol and tobacco, which have a drug-like effect, can also interact with estrogen. And watch for interactions between progestins and drugs such as steroids, antibiotics, and antidepressants.

Measuring Hormone Levels

Knowing how much estrogen you are producing can help you decide whether you need to supplement. Estrogen amount is assessed by measuring the level of follicle-stimulating hormone (FSH) in your blood, a standard lab test used to indicate the approach of menopause. FSH is produced by the pituitary gland in the brain and increases as estrogen production declines. A reading of below 20 IU/L (international units per liter) indicates that estrogen levels are normal, while a higher reading is a sign that a woman has begun the transition to menopause.

If you have this test done, be aware that a single reading is not a reliable indicator. A series of readings over months can vary dramatically. As a result, hormones may be prescribed when they are not needed, and medications may be prescribed when hormones are all that is needed. Single readings of estrogen and inhibin, another hormone produced by the ovaries, are also unreliable. A reliable indicator that a woman is in menopause is if levels of FSH are consistently elevated.

Having It Your Way

If you decide to take hormones, make a special effort to be aware of how they are affecting you. The goal is to take the least amount of medication that will still be effective in achieving the results you are after. Also experiment with the method of delivery. You may find it easier to take hormones in pill form, or you may prefer the convenience of using an estrogen patch. Watch for side effects. And if you decide to stop taking hormones, consult with your health care practitioner, who will probably advise you to stop gradually. Avoid an abrupt change that might trigger symptoms.

Women today have far more say about their own health care than in the past. Yet this freedom is hampered by a lack of understanding of the complex process of menopause, which, to some degree, is unique for each woman. This chapter can help you decide whether you want to take hormones, but the lack of sufficient research to date leaves some questions unanswered.

There will probably never be definitive advice to follow. The hormone decision must be made on an individual basis, but the more information you gather the better. Keep reading about menopause, talk to friends and health care providers, and remember to listen to your own thoughts and cues from your body. You are more of an expert on menopause than you may think!

CHAPTER TEN

Staying Healthy
as You Age

All too often, certain diseases that women are more likely to develop as they age are lumped together with the symptoms of menopause. These medical conditions include thyroid problems, urinary tract infections, incontinence, heart disease, and osteoporosis. A woman is not likely to develop such diseases just because she is female and menopausal. Having lower levels of estrogen, which occurs postmenopause, can increase a woman's risk of developing these conditions. However, a whole range of factors, including heredity and lifestyle, ultimately determine whether a woman ages without these diseases. These conditions can result from eating a nutrient-poor refined and processed foods diet, going without adequate exercise, living in a toxic environment, and leading a high-stress life.

The good news is that because the origins of these medical conditions are to a great extent rooted in lifestyle, you have considerable control over many of the risk factors. Let's take a look at each disease state in terms of symptoms, risk factors, what tests can tell you, and recommended therapies. The various approaches to natural healing incorporated in the Healthy Menopause Program can also help ensure long-term health. In some instances, hormone replacement therapy may be beneficial.

Thyroid Problems

If you have been feeling tired, even though you've been getting plenty of rest, you may have a sluggish thyroid—that is, hypothyroidism. The thyroid gland is a butterfly-shaped organ located on both sides of the windpipe and just below the Adam's apple. It produces thyroid hormones known as T_3 and T_4, and regulates the rate at which your body produces energy.

By age 50, one out of eight women naturally develop some degree of hypothyroidism, which is five to eight times more common in women than in men. Symptoms include chronic fatigue, painful and excessive menstrual periods in perimenopausal women, unexplained weight gain, depression, nervousness, poor memory, and lack of sexual desire—problems that are also typical of menopause. Other symptoms include dry, coarse hair, puffy face and eyes, slow heartbeat, brittle nails, constipation, and cold intolerance. If you have some of these symptoms, be sure to have your thyroid function tested so that the problems can be accurately treated.

Testing

You can ask your physician to order the standard thyroid test that measures thyroid-stimulating hormone (TSH). An elevated TSH indicates that the thyroid is not making enough thyroid hormone. Thyroid replacement supplements may be required to restore hormone balance. A low TSH indicates overactivity and may require special therapy.

Alternatively, you can administer your own thyroid test, which can be a more sensitive monitor of abnormal function. The best home test for hypothyroidism is taking your temperature randomly. Take your temperature many times throughout the day. If your temperature is consistently below 98°F, you probably are hypothyroid. Be sure to let your physician know your findings.

Natural Therapies

Normal thyroid function depends on having an adequate supply of iodine, a component of the hormones produced by the thyroid gland. While some foods, such as seafood, shellfish, and seaweed, are especially rich sources of iodine, other foods, if eaten raw, contain compounds (goitrogens) that can block iodine absorption. These include raw cauliflower, raw cabbage, raw turnips, raw brussels sprouts, raw kale, and soy products. However, you need to eat relatively large quantities of these to produce a significant effect. The chlorine and fluoride added to municipal water supplies can also interfere with thyroid hormone production. These chemicals block iodine receptor sites. Vitamin A, thiamin, and vitamin E, as well as the minerals manganese and zinc, are also required for thyroid health.

Herbs can be used in the treatment of hypothyroidism. These fall into the categories of bitters such as barberry, gentian root, and goldenseal, which act as stimulants, and nerve tonics such as damiana. Kelp, known to herbalists as bladderwrack, is a rich source of iodine, and is also commonly prescribed. Work with a trained herbalist to create an herbal formula that you can take as a tea. Possible herbs to include are bladderwrack, damiana or kola, nettles, oats, and wormwood.

Hormonal Therapy

For some women, thyroid function is affected by how much progesterone and estrogen are present in body tissues. Developing hypothyroidism may be linked to a decline in progesterone production, which occurs postmenopause. If you and your physician suspect the two conditions are associated, you may want to experiment with progesterone supplementation.

Another possibility is that excess estrogen has decreased the thyroid gland's intake of thyroid hormone. If you are taking estrogen replacement therapy and are troubled by hypothyroidism, you may want to reduce the dosage of your supplement to rule out ERT as the source of your thyroid problems.

Medications

The most common medication prescribed for hypothyroidism is levothyroxin, sold under the brand names Synthroid, Levothyroid, and Levoxyl. If you are taking one of these medications, be sure to have your physician regularly monitor your thyroid levels to make sure that the dosage is keeping your thyroid hormone levels within a target range. You should be aware that some studies link excessive doses of thyroid hormone with an increased risk of osteoporosis, as well as menstrual problems, hypertension, chest pain, palpitation, anxiety, and shortness of breath.

If these drugs are used long term, the body may lose its ability to produce thyroid hormone on its own. However, USP (United States Pharmacopeia) thyroid, a prescription drug derived from the thyroid glands of animals, which contains both T_3 and T_4, is not as likely to have this effect. About 60 to 70% of people taking this product regain their own hormone production once they discontinue the drug. The brand name for this product is Armour thyroid.

Urinary Tract Infection

One of the symptoms of menopause, discussed in Chapter 2, is the changes that occur in vaginal tissue, including thinning, drying, and a loss of elasticity, due to a decrease in estrogen production. Lowered estrogen levels affect the urinary tract in the same way. The urethra and bladder become drier, thinner, and lose muscle tone. As a result, tissue is more easily irritated and may become inflamed. Urinary flow may be impeded, setting the stage for infection as bacteria accumulate when the bladder does not empty completely. In fact, women post-menopause are about 15% more likely to develop urinary tract and bladder infections.

Urinating can produce a burning sensation in the urethra, and even if you urinate frequently, the feeling of needing to urinate may not go away. Fortunately, if you attend to cystitis as soon as symptoms appear, natural treatments can be very effective at reversing the infection.

Diet and Healing Foods

Both blueberries and cranberries are traditional food cures for cystitis. As bacteria multiply within the bladder, they cling to the bladder wall. However, a compound in the berries keeps the bacteria from sticking, so they are flushed out of the system in the urine. If you have cystitis, reach for some blueberries. Whole blueberries, now widely available, fresh in season and frozen out of season, are a far better choice. You can also process blueberries into a healing juice. A therapeutic dose is 1 to 1½ cups of juice a day.

Eating cranberries is a common home remedy for cystitis, but because cranberries are naturally very tart, cranberry products require a large amount of added sugar to make them palatable. This sugar can undermine the healing process. Bacteria feed on sugar and intake of quantities of sugar can weaken the immune system. Commercial cranberry juice is loaded with some form of sweetener. The ingredient list on the juice label may not include the word *sugar*, but you'll probably find terms such as *high-fructuose corn syrup*, *fruit juice concentrate*, and *evaporated cane juice*—all sources of sugar. You may, however, be able to find small bottles of cranberry juice concentrate in natural food stores. You can make a sugar-free drink by diluting this with water, but the result is still quite tart. If you must have cranberry, take it as an extract in tablet form.

Another way of flushing out bacteria is to drink plenty of fluids, which increases the amount of urine produced. Drink primarily filtered water and at least eight glasses a day.

Other healing foods include garlic and onions, both of which have natural antibacterial properties, and parsley, which is a diuretic and promotes urination.

Special Nutrients

Supporting the immune system with the nutritious way of eating recommended in the Healthy Menopause Program is important. Foods that deliver abundant vitamin C, vitamin A, and zinc—nutrients that support immune function—are especially beneficial. Include raw sweet peppers for vitamin C, orange-colored vegetables for vitamin A, and Brazil nuts and pumpkin seeds for zinc. Organic liver is also an excellent source of vitamin A, and oysters are a superb source of zinc. And when you are cooking, be sure to include garlic and onions.

To aggressively treat a urinary tract infection, the following supplements are recommended until symptoms subside:

Vitamin C: 500 to 1000 every 2 hours during waking hours daily

Vitamin A: 8000 IU daily

Zinc: 22 mg daily

Essential fatty acids: 1½ teaspoons flaxseed oil daily

Herbs

Certain medicinal herbs can be your allies, including dandelion, which is a diuretic; goldenseal, echinacea, and uva ursi, which fight infection; and motherwort, which tonifies tissues of the urinary tract. Here are some suggested dosages:

- DANDELION   3 cups daily of a decoction made with 2 to 3 teaspoons of the root in 1 cup of water or ½ to 1 teaspoon of the tincture daily
- GOLDENSEAL   2 cups a day taken as a tea, or ½ to 1 teaspoon of tincture three times a day
- ECHINACEA   3 cups daily of a decoction made with 1 to 2 teaspoons of the root in 1 cup of water, or ¼ to ¾ teaspoons of the tincture three times a day
- UVA URSI   1 teaspoon of tincture taken as a tea up to three times a day, or 1 cup of infusion up to three times a day (in sensitive persons, as little as ½ ounce can cause a toxic reaction such as ringing in the ears, nausea, vomiting, a feeling of suffocation, shortness of breath, convulsions, delirium, and collapse)
- MOTHERWORT   a maximum of 2 cups of tea daily or ½ teaspoon tincture up to twice daily

Exercise

Physical activity that increases the circulation of blood to the pelvic area will also promote healing. Aerobic exercise is an effective way of stimulating the blood.

Medications

Antibiotics are often prescribed to knock out a urinary tract infection. If you decide to go this route, be sure to also take some live-culture yogurt to replenish the beneficial bacteria in the urinary tract that can be destroyed by medication.

Incontinence

Changes in bladder tissue, including thinning, drying, and a lack of elasticity, can result in incontinence as well as urinary tract infection. With menopause and a decrease in estrogen production, pelvic and abdominal muscles that support the bladder can weaken. Women who have had children are particularly at risk.

Incontinence can be a source of great embarrassment. Probably for this reason the incidence of incontinence is underreported. Actually, about 30% of women over 40 become incontinent to one degree or another as they age.

You may find that coughing or simply laughing will cause you to suddenly and involuntarily release a small amount of urine. Incontinence can also be experienced as an urgent need to urinate that cannot be controlled. You may need to dash to the bathroom and may still not make it in time. In order to cope with these problems, women sometimes make drastic changes in the way they conduct their lives. Martha, who had been an executive secretary in a prominent law office for over 30 years, decided to no longer work in the office to manage her problem. She now works at home and telecommutes to continue her association with her longtime employer, but this change necessitated a drop in salary. Another woman who relished swimming in her neighbor's pool felt she had to give up this favorite form of relaxation for fear of becoming incontinent while exercising.

Fortunately, such drastic adjustments to incontinence can in many cases be avoided. You can take positive steps to lower the likelihood of being inconvenienced. The sooner you start the better.

Use It or Lose It

Practice the well-known Kegel exercises that strengthen the muscles that control urination: the pubococcygeal muscles that support the bladder and urethra. These are the muscles you use when you attempt to stop urination in midstream. A single sequence involves slowly tightening these muscles, holding them for a moment, and then relaxing them. A complete Kegel workout should include 50 to 100 repetitions. To correct incontinence, you will need to perform this set of exercises several times a day.

A Lady-like Approach

To stop incontinence in the short term, if you are seated you can always resort to crossing your legs! This move is socially acceptable and no one will realize your motive as you cough or laugh. This instinctive move can be quite effective and has even been confirmed in a scientific study.

Ignoring the Urge

Another approach to increasing the amount of urine you can hold is to resist the need to urinate even though you have the urge. Hold your bladder muscles tight through one or two urge spasms. This should stretch the bladder and increase its capacity.

Foods That Can Worsen Incontinence

Certain foods that can irritate the bladder and worsen incontinence include alcohol, beverages that contain caffeine, spicey foods, dairy foods, acidic foods such as coffee and colas, acidic produce such as citrus, strawberries, and tomatoes, and sugar.

Treating Incontinence with Herbs

Incontinence can in some cases be brought under control through the use of herbs even when it occurs because the sphincter muscles of the bladder are weak or the nerves controlling bladder function are impaired. One effective herbal mixture is horsetail, sweet sumach, and agrimony, taken as a tea. Consult with an experienced herbalist to develop an herbal formula suited to your specific needs.

Other Avenues of Treatment

A basic way to gain more control over the urge to urinate is to drink lots of water so that your bladder fills, and then when you have the urge to urinate, practice resisting this. Resist only briefly, but try to lengthen the time you can hold back the urge as you repeat this exercise. Alternatively, you might want to experiment with timed toileting, pacing when urination occurs throughout the day.

And some women find biofeedback beneficial. Biofeedback involves learning to regulate normally unconscious bodily functions, such as holding urine in the bladder, to acquire voluntary control over these. If biofeedback is practiced regularly, a degree of continence can be restored.

Medical intervention is another option. Detrol, Ditropan, and Cystospaz are prescribed to reduce the urge to go all the time. However, these medications must be carefully chosen and the effects of taking them must be monitored closely, as they can cause serious side effects, including glaucoma and bladder retention.

And if none of these approaches is beneficial and you find incontinence is disrupting your life, you may also want to consider corrective surgery as a final option. This usually involves suspending the bladder and tightening the attachments to the bladder that help support it within the abdominal cavity. Along with this procedure, many gynecologists also highly recommend a hysterectomy in which the uterus is removed. As a woman ages, the uterus is less able to resist the pull of gravity and its position drops, also dragging down the bladder. This movement alters the angle between the bladder and the urethra (the canal through which urine flows from the bladder to the outside), which interferes with normal urination.

Heart Disease

Younger women have much less of a risk of heart disease than men of the same age, but after menopause a woman's risk can increase dramatically. In fact, heart attack, stroke, and other diseases of the heart and blood vessels are the leading causes of death among American women. About 9 million women of all ages suffer from heart disease, and every year a half million women suffer heart attacks. Despite these statistics, heart disease is still more commonly associated with males. One reason may be that until recently most research on heart disease studied male subjects almost exclusively. Research is now in progress to examine heart disease in women, but conclusive results, comparable to what is known about the disease in men, are still years away.

One avenue of research actively being pursued is the effect of estrogen on heart health. In that a woman's risk increases after menopause, scientists and many physicians have begun to treat heart problems as an estrogen deficiency disease. Using this line of reasoning, hormone replacement therapy becomes the preventive measure of choice. Indeed, estrogen does appear to help keep undersirable LDL (low-density lipoprotein) levels low and desirable HDL (high-density lipoprotein) levels high. There is also mixed evidence that estrogen lowers blood fats, which play a role in heart problems. Estrogen also reduces changes in the arteries that increase the risk of cardiovascular disease. However, how to interpret these findings is under question.

Heart health requires more support than hormone replacement therapy (HRT). Even if HRT helps prevent cardiovascular disease, it alone is useless unless factors that promote heart disease are also controlled. These include poor diet, lack of exercise, excess weight, excessive intake of caffeine and alcohol, smoking, high blood pressure, and diabetes. Whether or not you are taking hormones, you still have to take good care of your health.

For long-term heart health, there is no substitute for wise lifestyle choices, and following the advice on diet and exercise in the Six-Step Healthy Menopause Program is a good place to start.

Healthy Fats

High intake of saturated fats, such as butter and the fat in meats, is associated with heart disease. This fact has been well publicized and most women worried about heart health avidly avoid saturated fat and other types of fat as well. Herein lies the problem. Some fats benefit the heart and are necessary for the normal functioning of tissues and organs. The monounsaturates found in olive oil and almonds help lower cholesterol, and the omega-3 essential fatty acids present in fish and walnuts help transport cholesterol from the arteries to the liver where it is broken down and then excreted By dramatically cutting back on fat intake in general, you risk not taking in sufficient quantities of these healing oils.

Consuming a very low-fat diet can even lead to hormone imbalance, which can bring on menopausal symptoms, including fatigue, depression, and dry vaginal tissues and skin. And low-fat food products are often high in sugar, which can upset glucose metabolism associated with heart disease. A low-fat diet may also be low in protein, which is needed to support adrenal function, including the production of sex hormones.

Cholesterol Worries

The cholesterol in your diet is not likely to raise your blood cholesterol levels as much as the saturated fat you eat. In addition, research indicates that oxidized cholesterol and not cholesterol itself is the culprit in heart disease. For this reason, the antioxidant nutrients, vitamin C, vitamin E, beta-carotene, and selenium, are now routinely recommended for their heart-protective benefits.

Fiber also lowers cholesterol. Eating five servings a day of fruits and vegetables, the minimum intake recommended, is a good way to start. Studies show that whole grains are also heart-healthy foods. According to an editorial in 1999, in the *American Journal of Clinical Nutrition*, which reviewed several studies, whole-grain intake reduces the risk of coronary artery disease, as well as hypertension, a risk factor for heart disease. These benefits are likely to be due to various components of the grains—the fiber as well as the complex carbohydrates, vitamins, minerals, and phytoestrogens.

Special Healing Foods

Three delicious flavorings—garlic, onion, and ginger—are heart-friendly foods. Garlic is a traditional healing food prescribed to prevent blood clots. Onion lowers blood pressure and ginger stimulates circulation.

A Word on Hypertension

Reducing sodium in your diet can help lower blood pressure. However, sodium does not cause high blood pressure, and if you have normal blood pressure, you have no reason to avoid salt. Rather, focus on your potassium intake, the mineral that is plentiful in bananas and potatoes. Low potassium intake, coupled with high sodium intake, is linked to high blood pressure.

Exercise

Even moderate exercise can benefit the heart. Go out of your way to work into your schedule at least a half hour of some form of exercise three times a week. Take a stroll in your neighborhood or do some heavy gardening. Opt for stairs rather than an elevator when you can. You don't have to work up a big sweat to benefit. And stress-reducing forms of exercise such as yoga, with its regulated breathing, help relax the body and have been proven to lower blood pressure.

Herbal Supplements

Hawthorne berries benefit the heart in a variety of ways: reducing cholesterol, lowering blood pressure, reducing angina attacks, and preventing cholesterol from depositing on arterial walls. Enjoy 1 to 2 cups of hawthorne tea a day, or ½ to 1 teaspoon of tincture of hawthorne three times daily.

Bromelain, an enzyme derived from pineapple, can break down plaque, and lower blood pressure and blood clotting. Supplement with bromelain capsules between meals.

Tests

Several standard tests are given to assess heart health. These include measuring blood pressure, cholesterol, and triglycerides.

A test of blood pressure measures the force of blood as it presses against the walls of the arteries. Systolic pressure is the force of the blood while the heart is pumping and diastolic pressure is the force of the blood with the heart at rest. Use the following chart to interpret your results:

Resting	Systolic	Diastolic
Normal	Below 130	Below 85
High normal	130–139	85–89
Hypertension	140 or higher	90 or higher

Cholesterol is measured by taking a blood sample. The only really telling cholesterol readings are HDL and LDL individually. Total cholesterol is actually meaningless without the other numbers. Good readings are high HDL and low LDL, regardless of what these two figures total. This is true especially for women with only minimal risk factors for heart disease. Here are figures against which to measure your score.

Total Cholesterol	*HDL*	*LDL*
DESIRABLE		
Less than 200	35 or higher	Less than 100
BORDERLINE		
200–239	35	100–130
NOT DESIRABLE		
Over 240	Less than 35	130 or higher

A third test measures triglyceride or blood fat levels. This is more predictive of heart disease in women than in men, but a high triglyceride reading by itself may not be a risk factor. For health, you need a triglyceride reading of under 180 mg/dl (milligrams per deciliter).

Osteoporosis

Another degenerative disease often linked to menopause is osteoporosis. As estrogen and progesterone production decline, bone loss accelerates. However, the reasons for the onset of osteoporosis are more complex. Lifestyle also plays a vitally important role.

In osteoporosis, bones become abnormally thin as the very

structure of the bone starts to break down. Bone fracture can result. Between 7 and 8 million Americans, 80% women, have some form of osteoporosis. Each year there are about 1.5 million cases of related fractures of the wrist, spine, or hip. Hip fractures make up 25% of total fractures and can be particularly debilitating. Half of hip fracture patients lose the ability to live independently, and 20% of those suffering from such fractures die within the first year.

Bone Is Ever-changing

Your bones are made up of living tissue that is continuously being reshaped. There is compact or cortical bone, which seems solid and hard, and trabecular bone, which is spongy and lighter. The shafts of long bones such as your legs and arms are made up of compact bone. The end of the long bones, spinal vertebrae, ribs, heel bones, and jaw are comprised of the spongy trabecular bone. Both types of bones undergo remodeling, cell by cell. Osteoclasts—specialized cells—break down worn out bone, while osteoblasts build back the old segment with new bone. As much as one-fifth of your skeleton is replaced each year.

Bones reach their peak density between a woman's mid-20s and late 30s. Then, in her early 40s, a shift in the natural process of the breaking down of bone begins to outpace the bone-building process. Gradual bone loss of 1% or less per year becomes a normal part of aging. This process accelerates with menopause for a period of 4 or 5 years before returning to a slower rate. As production of estrogen and progesterone decline, bones become more porous. The illustration shows typical changes in bone composition.

Especially if you have a family history of osteoporosis, as you enter perimenopause you may want to ask your physician to order a bone density test for a baseline reading.

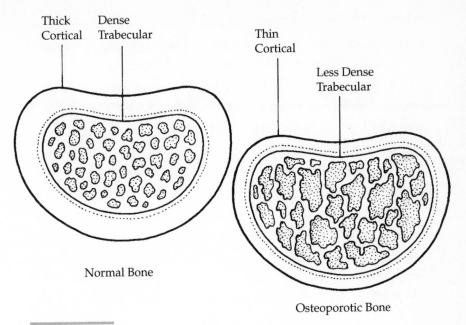

Thick Cortical Dense Trabecular

Thin Cortical

Less Dense Trabecular

Normal Bone

Osteoporotic Bone

Bone Density

Testing for Bone Density

Bone mineral density is best measured by dual-energy x-ray absorptiometer, which is given the acronym DEXA. A full DEXA screening focuses on the central bones of the body and is particularly appropriate for women who have obvious risk factors for osteoporosis. Advanced equipment models offer computer processing of the information, enabling faster scans and bilateral femur evaluation with a rapid lumbar spine assessment.

Alternatively, bone status can be screened through a minimal DEXA study of the heel, with further screening done only if required. Facilities that offer heel DEXAs often offer these at a reduced cost, which is deferred completely if the full DEXA is recommended and performed within a limited time period.

The density of bones in the heel can also be assessed using ultrasound. However, this is appropriate for screening purposes only.

Bone mineral density is expressed as a *t*-score, which represents the difference in standard deviation (SD) when compared with peak bone mass. A Z-score is the difference of the subject's SD compared with healthy age-matched controls. Osteoporosis is indicated when the SD is –2.5 or lower. Fracture risk increases 1½ to 2½ times for each SD of an individual's bone mass below peak bone mass.

However, bone mineral density is not the only predictor of fractures. Increasingly, muscle strength and functional agility are being factored in as well. Only at advanced levels of osteoporosis is a woman at risk for spontaneous vertebral fracture or a fracture from such simple activities as coughing. At moderate levels of bone loss, her risk of falling must be taken into account. That is, a feeble and wobbly woman with a bone density reading of –1.0 is conceivably at greater risk of fracture that a sturdy, agile woman with a bone density of –2.0.

Note: The only way you can really know if your bone is becoming more porous is to have your bones tested several times. As you enter perimenopause, have your bone density assessed annually. Comparing the results over the years gives you a way to measure your own individual rate of bone loss. If you naturally have less dense bones, a single test can make it appear that you are developing osteoporosis when you are not.

Osteoporosis and Hormones

Taking estrogen can cut back on the rapid bone loss associated with menopause and can significantly cut down on hip fractures during this time. However, if a woman stops taking estrogen, her rate of bone loss will increase to that typical of the first stages of menopause. Alternatively, a woman can continue to take estrogen for the rest of her life, but this increases her risk of other medical conditions as described in Chapter 9. In addition, supplemental estrogen does not build bone but simply helps prevent its loss.

In contrast, there is evidence that progesterone, which also declines at menopause, can stimulate the bone-building cells, the osteoblasts. A small but impressive study conducted by Dr. John Lee demonstrated the effectiveness of supplementing with natural progesterone to rebuild bone.

Standard protocols for preventing and treating osteoporosis include a combination of therapies that include hormone replacement as well as supplementing with calcium and vitamin D. Occasionally, the hormone calcitonin is also prescribed. Various studies have tested combination therapies. In one, published in 1990 in *Obstetrics and Gynecology*, estrone sulfate given in a daily dosage of 0.625 milligrams, combined with 1000 milligrams of elemental calcium, was the minimum effective dosage to prevent loss of spinal bone mineral density in postmenopausal women over a 12-month period. In another study, published in 1994 in the *Annals of Internal Medicine*, calcium alone significantly retarded bone loss from the femoral neck and improved calcium balance in recently postmenopausal women. However, in the same study, a combination of estrogen, progesterone, and calcium proved even more effective.

Each woman, working with her physician, needs to design a treatment plan suited to her needs, based on her risk of osteoporosis as well as other diseases. But whatever course a woman chooses, following a lifestyle that supports bone health is essential, including proper diet and exercise.

Osteoporosis and Lifestyle

Although osteoporosis is most prevalent among older women, the disease appears to be more linked to lifestyle than it is to age and gender. Osteoporosis is far more common in Western cultures such as those of the British Isles and North America, where refined and processed foods make up the majority of most meals and many women do not receive sufficient exercise. In countries such as India, significant bone lose with associated bone fractures is less prevalent. In such cultures, the diet is still made up of predominantly unprocessed foods and women's daily activities include more weight-bearing physical activity.

Osteoporosis and Acidic Foods

In Western societies, highly acidic foods are consumed at every meal. If such foods are not kept in balance with alkaline ingredients, eating this way can lead to a depletion of the mineral content of bones. Some acidic foods such as vinaigrette salad dressing can be identified by taste, but the majority of acidic foods are not quickly recognized. These include white flour, white sugar, meats, fatty foods such as french fries, tomatoes, dairy foods, coffee, tea, cola, and alcohol. The chemical reactions involved in converting these foods to energy result in the formation of acidic substances that can accumulate in body tissues. This in turn can disrupt and slow normal body function. Chemical reactions can only take place in a cellular environment with a precise balance between acids and alkalines. When the system becomes too acidic, the body will draw alkaline minerals such as calcium from bones in order to continue to function. This ongoing process eventually takes its toll on skeletal strength.

To offset these acidifying tendencies of the North American diet, make sure you eat plenty of alkalizing foods at each meal including vegetables, fruits, whole grains, and legumes such as beans, lentils, and peas. Rely on filtered water to quench your thirst, not colas that contain sugar, caffeine, and phosphorus, all of which tend to pull mineral from bone.

Avoid habitual intake of alcohol, coffee, and black tea. High alcohol intake is associated with osteoporosis. And if you enjoy having coffee or tea, make these beverages occasional treats. Sipping on these caffeinated drinks throughout the day is a good way to increase mineral loss. A 1993 study, published in the *Journal of Nutrition*, demonstrated that oral doses of caffeine increased the urinary excretion of calcium and magnesium. However, even decaffeinated coffee and tea place demands on bone mineral as these beverages are highly acidic.

Eating a Varied Diet for Nutrients

Calcium, so heavily promoted for preventing osteoporosis, is only one of many nutrients needed to build bone. Bone also requires magnesium, manganese, phosphorus, vitamin K, folic acid, boron, vitamin B_6, zinc, strontium, copper, silicon, vitamin C, and vitamin D. In a 1986 study, published in the *American Journal of Clinical Nutrition*, high consumption levels of phosphorus, zinc, and folate, as well as calcium, correlated with slower bone loss.

Eating a variety of fruits, vegetables, legumes, grains, nuts, and seeds can help ensure that your diet includes the full range of these nutrients. Make an effort to regularly consume magnesium-rich foods such as beans, brown rice, and green vegetables. The absorption of calcium depends upon having adequate magnesium intake. Good food sources of calcium include dairy products such as live-bacteria yogurt, unrefined whole grains including cornmeal and whole wheat, beans, dark leafy greens like kale and bok choy, fruit including figs and papaya, hazelnuts, sesame seeds, canned fish with bones, and blackstrap molasses.

CALCIUM AND DAIRY FOODS

Many women rely on dairy products as their calcium source, but these foods can be counterproductive. In fact, in

North America, Britain, and Scandinavia, where osteoporosis is most common, intake of dairy foods, including calcium-rich milk, is especially high.

- A dairy food such as milk is a high-protein food, which tends to acidify the system and encourage bone loss.

- Milk and cheese are high in fat, implicated in heart disease and cancer. And eating low-fat dairy foods is not a solution, because now you have an even more concentrated source of acidifying protein.

- Dairy foods are also very low in magnesium.

- Most commercial milk and other dairy foods contain added hormones given to cows to increase production, as well as traces of pesticides that can behave like estrogen once they are consumed.

If you enjoy dairy products, choose high-quality organic foods, free of added hormones. Yogurt is good because it provides friendly bacteria that benefit digestive health.

Taking Supplements

If you are premenopausal, the standard recommendation is 1000 milligrams of calcium a day. This is also the recommendation for postmenopausal women who are taking estrogen. However, if you are postmenopausal and not on estrogen, the standard recommendation increases to 1500 milligrams a day. These relatively high amounts of calcium help compensate for the effects of the acidic Western diet. In non-Western cultures, calcium intake as low as 200 to 475 milligrams a day appears to be sufficient to maintain bone health, an amount easily obtained through diet. The Bantu women of South Africa consume calcium within this range and yet osteoporosis is rare.

Calcium citrate appears to be a well-absorbed form of calcium in older women who may have reduced production of stomach acid, which is necessary for absorbing calcium. Another form of calcium is microcrystalline hydroxyapatate concentrate (MCHC). Studies show that MCHC is particularly effective in building bone.

Whatever supplement you take, calcium is best absorbed if taken in divided doses throughout the day, accompanied by food.

Magnesium intake should be based on the amount of calcium being supplemented because these two nutrients work together. If dietary intake is low, you may need to take as much magnesium as calcium. Other recommended dosages are as follows:

Vitamin B_6: 50 to 100 mg per day.

Folic acid: 400 to 1000 mcg per day.

Vitamin C: 1000 to 3000 mg per day.

Vitamin D: not to exceed a total of 800 IU per day without professional supervision. Amounts higher than those found in a good multivitamin-mineral are generally needed by older people who get very little sunlight.

Boron: 2 to 4 mg per day.

Copper: 2 to 4 mg per day.

Silica: 100 to 1000 mg per day.

Manganese: 10 to 15 mg per day.

Zinc: 20 to 25 mg per day.

Exercise

Weight-bearing exercise, as described in Chapter 7, is essential for bone health. The force of impact or weight on a bone triggers minerals to be deposited on bone in an effort to withstand this stress. In an informal study of highway workers using pneumatic drills to remove asphalt, the bones of these men were found to be exceptionally well developed and strong although exposed to wear and tear throughout the day. By contrast, it is well known that invalids, restricted to bed, quickly lose bone strength.

Herbs

Although herbs are not as useful as diet and exercise at preventing osteoporosis, certain herbs are good sources of calcium and sometimes are included in herbal formulas designed for menopause. Look for the following: chickweed, comfrey, dandelion greens, mustard greens, nettle, oat straw, and watercress. Herbs that help balance hormones, described in Chapter 6, are also good choices.

Stress and Osteoporosis

Stress can weaken bones in two ways. It can acidify the system, just as diet can. As a consequence, minerals are drawn from the bones to contribute alkalinity and restore pH balance. Stress also overworks the adrenals, the glands that manage the stress response. Postmenopause, the adrenal glands are an important source of estrogen precursors that add significantly to a woman's supply of this hormone. Reducing stress keeps adrenals strong and maximizes estrogen production, which in turn supports skeletal health.

Medications

Fosamax is a new nonhormonal, bisphosphonate drug approved in 1995 by the Food and Drug Administration for the treatment of osteoporosis. It has only been studied for a few years but appears to halt spinal bone loss. However, because this drug works by interfering with the bone-remodeling process, it is not clear whether it may also prevent worn-out bone from being replaced.

Glossary

Adrenal glands. Small, pyramid-shaped glands situated on top of each kidney that secrete various substances, among which are the steroid hormones androgen, estrogen, and progesterone.

Antioxidant. Substance that prevents oxidation or inhibits reactions promoted by oxygen.

Artificial hormones. Hormones derived from plant substances that have a chemical configuration differing from the hormones that a woman's body naturally makes.

Bioflavonoid. Constituent of the vitamin C complex.

Blood-sugar level. Amount of glucose (sugar) circulating in the bloodstream.

Calcium balance. Net processes in which calcium enters the body (through the diet) and leaves the body (through sweat, urine, and feces).

Cervix. Narrow lower end of the uterus that extends into the vagina.

Collagen. Protein that is the supportive component of bone, connective tissue, cartilage, and skin.

Corpus luteum.   The small yellow endocrine structure that develops in the ovary after ovulation, the cells of which produce progesterone and estrogen as well as other hormones.

Endocrine glands.   Glands that manufacture hormones, and release them into the bloodstream.

Enzyme.   Protein capable of producing or accelerating a specific biochemical reaction at body temperature.

Essential fatty acids.   Healthy fats that the body is unable to produce and must be provided by the diet.

Estrogen.   Female hormone responsible for stimulating the development of female secondary sex characteristics.

Fibroids.   Fibrous, noncancerous growths most commonly found in or on the uterus.

Follicle-stimulating hormone (FSH).   A hormone produced by the pituitary gland that stimulates development of follicles in the ovaries and the secretion of estrogen.

Free radicals.   Highly reactive molecular fragments, generally harmful to the body.

Glucose.   Simple sugar that is the usual form in which carbohydrates exist in the bloodstream.

Glycogen.   Principal form in which a carbohydrate is stored in the body for ready conversion into energy; found in the liver and in muscle tissue in particular.

HDL cholesterol.   High-density lipoprotein; the form of cholesterol associated with a lower risk of heart disease.

Hormone.   Substance produced in one part of the body and carried in the blood to another part of the body, where it chemically stimulates that part to increase or decrease functional activity or the secretion of another hormone.

Hysterectomy.   Surgical removal of the uterus (a radical hysterectomy includes removal of the uterus, cervix, ovaries, fallopian tubes, and sometimes lymph nodes near the ovaries).

LDL cholesterol.   Low-density lipoprotein; the undesirable form of cholesterol associated with a greater risk of heart disease.

Luteinizing hormone (LH).   Hormone produced by the pituitary (a large surge of this hormone in each menstrual cycle precedes ovulation by 12 to 24 hours).

Metabolism.   Sum of chemical changes; the building up or destruction of cells that takes place in the body.

Natural hormones.   Hormones made in a laboratory that have the same chemical configuration as the hormones produced by a woman's body.

Neurotransmitter.   Substance that transmits nerve impulses across a synapse; brain chemical that is involved in carrying messages to and from the brain.

Ovary.   One of two female organs containing the eggs and the cells that produce the female hormones estrogen and progesterone.

Ovulation.   Process during which a mature egg is released from the ovary.

Oxidation.   Process of combining with oxygen.

Pituitary gland.   Small, oval organ at the base of the brain that produces many important hormones (particularly FSH and LH) and has been called the "master gland."

Progesterone.   A steroid hormone responsible for the changes in the endometrium in the second half of the menstrual cycle preparatory for implantation, development of the maternal placenta, and development of the mammary glands. Used to treat menstrual disorders, among other problems.

Prostaglandins.   One of several compounds formed from essential fatty acids and whose activities affect the nervous, circulatory, and reproductive systems and metabolism. Research indicates that a type of prostaglandin is implicated in muscular contractions and menstrual cramps.

Trans-fatty acid.   An unnatural synthetic fat that has a twist in its structure; heating polyunsaturated fats to high temperatures, in cooking and in the process of hydrogenation to make margarine, causes trans-fatty acids to form.

Sources

Chapter 2

Haines, C. J., et al. A prospective study of the frequency of acute menopausal symptoms in Hong Kong Chinese women. *Maturitas* 1994; 18:175–181.

Hilton, E., et al. Ingestion of yogurt containing *Lactobacillus acidophilus* as prophylaxis for candidal vaginitis. *Annals of Internal Medicine* 1992; 116(5):353–357.

Kronenberg, Fredi. Hot flashes: epidemiology and physiology. *Annals of the New York Academy of Sciences* 1990; 592:52–86.

Ley, Christopher J., et al. Sex and menopause associated changes in body-fat distribution. *American Journal of Clinical Nutrition* 1992; 55:950–954.

Chapter 4

Adlercreutz, Herman, et al. Urinary excretion of lignans and isoflavonoid phytoestrogens in Japanese men and women consuming a traditional Japanese diet. *American Journal of Clinical Nutrition* 1991; 54:1093–1100.

Chapter 5

Health Academy. *Prevention Magazine* 1993; 73–80.

Smith, Bob L. Organic foods vs supermarket foods: element levels. *Journal of Applied Nutrition* 1993; 45(1):35–39.

Wilcox, G., et al. Oestrogenic effects of plant foods in post-menopausal women. *British Medical Journal* 1990; 301(6757):905–906.

Chapter 6

Ornish, D., et al. Intensive lifestyle changes for reversal of coronary heart disease. *Journal of the American Medical Association* 1999; 281(15):1380.

Chapter 7

Freedman, R. R., and S. Woodward. Behavioral treatment of menopausal hot flashes: evaluation by ambulatory monitoring. *American Journal of Obstetrics and Gynecology* 1992; 167(2):436–439.

Prince, R. L., et al. Prevention of postmenopausal osteoporosis. A comparative study of exercise, calcium supplementation, and hormone-replacement therapy. *New England Journal of Medicine* 1991; 325(17):1189–1195.

Chapter 8

Swartzman, L. C., et al. Impact of stress on objectively recorded menopausal hot flashes and on flush report bias. *Health Psychology* 1990; 9(5):529–545.

Chapter 9

Hulley, S., et al. Randomized trial of estrogen plus progestin for secondary prevention of coronary heart disease in postmenopausal women. Heart and Estrogen/progestin Replacement Study (HERS) Research Group. *Journal of the American Medical Association* 1998; 280(7):605–613.

Mathews, Karen A., et al. Prior to use of estrogen replacement therapy, are users healthier than nonusers? *American Journal of Epidemiology* 1996; 143:971–978.

Schairer, C., et al. Menopausal estrogen and estrogen-progestin replacement therapy and breast cancer risk. *Journal of the American Medical Association* 2000; 283(4):485–491.

Writing Group for the PEPI Trial. Effects of estrogen/progestin regimens on heart disease risk factors in post-menopausal women. The Postmenopausal Estrogen/Progestin Interventions (PEPI) Trial. *Journal of the American Medical Association* 1995; 274(21):1676.

Chapter 10

Aloia, J. F., et al. Calcium supplementation with and without hormone replacement therapy to prevent postmenopausal bone loss. *Annals of Internal Medicine* 1994; 120(2):97–103.

Freudenheim, J. I., et al. Relationships between usual nutrient intake and bone-mineral content of women 35–65 years of age: longitudinal and cross-sectional analysis. *American Journal of Clinical Nutrition* 1986; 44(6):863–876.

Genant, H. K., et al. Effect of estrone sulfate on post-menopausal bone loss. *Obstetrics and Gynecology* 1990; 76(4):579–584.

Hulley, S., et al. Randomized trial of estrogen plus progestin for secondary prevention of coronary heart disease in post-menopausal women. Heart and Estrogen/progestin Replacement Study (HERS) Research Group. *Journal of the American Medical Association* 1998; 280(7):605–613.

Lee, J. R. Is natural progesterone the missing link in osteoporosis prevention and treatment? *Medical Hypothesis* 1991; 35(4):316–318.

Massey, L. K., and S. J.Whiting. Caffeine, urinary calcium, calcium metabolism and bone. *Journal of Nutrition* 1993; 123(9):1611–1614.

Resources

Health Organizations
and Information Resources

American Botanical Council
P.O. Box 144345
Austin, TX 78714
1-512-926-4900
Fax: 1-512-926-2345
e-mail: abc@herbalgram.org
www.herbalgram.org
Authoritative source of information on the medicinal uses of
   herbs.

American Menopause Foundation, Inc.
Empire State Building
350 Fifth Avenue, Suite 2822
New York, NY 10118
1-212-714-2398
Fax: 1-212-714-1252
Founder Marie Lugano operates a national network of support groups that deal with alternative treatments, among
   other issues. The organization also publishes a newsletter.

Bastyr University
Continuing Education Department
14500 Juanita Drive NE
Bothell, WA 98011
1-425-602-3152

The focus of Bastyr University is natural medicine, and information on this subject is available through several avenues: The library has bibliographies on women's health and the bookstore carries related titles and has a mail-order service. The Bastyr clinic can be contacted for questions and dispensary-related items and is reached at 1-206-632-0354.

Center for Science in the Public Interest
Americans for Safe Food Project
1875 Connecticut Avenue NW, Suite 300
Washington, DC 20009-5728
1-202-332-9110, ext. 384

You can obtain a list of organic mail-order suppliers and hormone-free beef suppliers, both supermarket chains and mail-order home delivery, from this organization.

DES Action USA
1615 Broadway, #510
Oakland, CA 94612
1-800-DES-9288 or 1-510-465-4011

A national consumer organization representing DES mothers, daughters, and sons. Dedicated to informing the public and health professions about the effects of DES and what can be done about them and to promoting DES research. Offers physician referrals, special publications, and a quarterly newsletter, *DES Action Voice*. If you were born between 1938 and 1971, you may have been exposed to DES and have an increased risk for some cancers.

Eden Acres
Organic Network
12100 Lima Center Road
Clinton, MI 49236-9618
1-517-456-4288
Organic Network, a division of Eden Acres, offers a 150-page international directory and local statewide directories of suppliers of organic meats, poultry, fruits, and vegetables.

Herb Research Foundation
1007 Pearl Street, Suite 200
Boulder, CO 80302
1-303-449-2265
The foundation supplies an information packet on herbs for a small fee. Write the organization for a free brochure.

National Association for Continence
Box 8310
Spartanburg, SC 29305
1-800-BLADDER
Fax: 1-803-579-7902
Offers information on bladder-control problems and the health care professionals who treat them.

National Black Women's Health Project
1211 Connecticut Avenue NW, Suite 310
Washington, DC 20036
Fax: 1-202-833-8709
Dedicated to reducing health care problems prevalent among African Americans, such as cervical cancer, diabetes, hypertension, obesity, and teenage pregnancy.

National Osteoporosis Foundation
P.O. Box 96173
Washington, DC 20077-7456
1-202-223-2226
NOF offers quite a lot for its membership, which includes a
60-page handbook, *Boning Up on Osteoporosis*, a quarterly
newsletter, and an invitation to contact the National Osteoporosis Patient Information Center.

National Women's Health Resource Center
2425 L Street NW, 3rd floor
Washington, DC 20037
1-202-293-6045
National clearinghouse for women's health information.

North American Menopause Society (NAMS)
Department of Ob/Gyn, University Hospitals of Cleveland
2074 Abingdon Road
Cleveland, OH 44106
1-216-844-3348
e-mail: nams@apk.net
www.menopause.org
NAMS is the leading scientific nonprofit organization for
menopause information. Members receive *Menopause*, a scientific journal, and *Menopause Management*, a journal for clinicians. The organization also offers a free 48-page
Menopause Guidebook for $5 postage and a book for those
who have experienced an induced menopause. The Web site
contains lots of links for clinicians and those interested in
health care information.

Wellspring for Women
1-303-443-0321
The organization offers phone consultations with licensed
nurse practitioners who can answer questions about herbal

remedies and natural hormones. They can also put you in touch with doctors who can prescribe them. The staff can discuss conventional hormone therapy. There is a fee for a minimum 45-minute consultation.

Locating Alternative Health Professionals

The following organizations can supply a directory of U.S. practitioners:

American Association of Naturopathic Physicians
P.O. Box 20386
Seattle, WA 98112

American Institute of Homeopathy
1585 Glencoe Street, #44
Denver, CO 80220

American Society of Acupuncture and Oriental Medicine
1424 16th Street NW, #501
Washington, DC 20036
1-202-265-2287

International Foundation for Homeopathy
2366 Eastlake Avenue East, Suite 322
Seattle, WA 98102
1-206-323-7610

National Academy of Environmental Medicine
P.O. Box 16106
Denver, CO 80216
1-303-622-9755

National Center for Homeopathy
801 North Fairfax Street, Suite 306
Alexandria, VA 22314
1-703-548-7790

Health Resource Phone Numbers

American Cancer Society 1-800-ACS-2345

American Heart Association 1-800-242-8721

Endometriosis Association 1-800-922-3636

HERS Foundation (Hysterectomy Education Resources &
    Services) 1-610-667-7757

National Alliance of Breast Cancer Organizations
    1-212-889-0606

National Cancer Institute's Cancer Information Service
    1-800-4-CANCER

Y-Me Hotline Breast Cancer Information and Support
    1-800-221-2141

Newletters/Publications

A Friend Indeed
P.O. Box 260
Pembina, ND 58271
e-mail: afi@pangea.ca
This research-based eight-page newsletter is the oldest
    menopause newsletter in North America. Each issue
    includes a feature article, often written by a nationally
    known expert in the field, along with letters from women
    and up-to-date research news.

Crone Chronicles
P.O. Box 81
Kelly, WY 83011
1-307-733-5409

The mission of this 10-year-old 80-page quarterly, "to activate the archetype of the Crone within contemporary culture," emerged from the belief that stories from Our Inner Crones need to be told. If wisdom can be gleaned from one's own experience, then this magazine is full of the wisdom that comes when we engage in conscious aging. *Crone Chronicles* was featured on *Good Morning America* in February 1999 and was a finalist for an Utne Reader annual award in 1998.

Environmental Nutrition
P.O. Box 42051
Palm Coast, FL 32142-0451
1-800-829-5384

This reputable publication presents research news about nutrition and supplements as related to health issues.

Harvard Women's Health Watch
P.O. Box 420068
Palm Coast, FL 32142-0068
1-800-829-5921

A potpourri of late-breaking information presented for the laywoman.

Health Hunter
Center for the Improvement of Human Functioning
    International
3100 North Hillside Avenue
Wichita, KS 67219
1-316-682-3100

A trustworthy source of information on all aspects of health, with a focus on the role of diet and specific nutrients in preventing various ailments and disease.

Health Wisdom for Women
7811 Montrose Road
Potomac, MD 20854
1-808-804-0935
Newsletter authored by Christiane Northrup, M.D., author of
    the best-selling authoritative book on female health,
    Women's Bodies, Women's Wisdom.

Menopause News
2074 Union Street
San Francisco, CA 94128
1-800-241-MENO
www.well.com/-mnews
Another well-researched newsletter focusing on specific topics
    along with book reviews and other information of interest to
    midlife women.

Midlife Wellness Center for Climacteric Studies
University of Florida
901 NW 8th Avenue, Suite B
Gainesville, FL 32601
Publishes a quarterly journal on menopause and aging.

National Women's Health Network
514 10th Street NW, Suite 400
Washington, DC 20004
1-202-347-1140
A membership education and advocacy organization that pub-
    lishes a newsletter and packets of information on ERT/HRT
    and alternative treatments.

Older Women's League (OWL)
666 11th Street NW, Suite 700
Washington, DC 20001-4512
1-202-783-6686
A membership and advocacy organization that publishes a
  newsletter.

Women's Health Advocate
P.O. Box 420089
Palm Coast, FL 32142
Update of research of interest to women, with brief but timely,
  well-written, and useful information.

Women's Health Connection
P.O. Box 6338
Madison, WI 53716-0338
1-800-366-6632
This educational division of Women's International Pharmacy
  publishes a bimonthly newsletter on menopause, premenstrual syndrome, and other hormone-related disorders.

Worst Pills, Best Pills
1600 20th Street NW
Washington, DC 20009
Published by Public Citizen Health Research Group,
  cofounded in 1971 by Ralph Nader and Sidney Wolfe,
  M.D., to give consumers more control over decisions that
  affect their health.

Web Pages

Check out these Web pages to research a multitude of aspects of female health and to join supportive communities of women in cyberspace.

cpmcnet.columbia.edu/dept/rosenthal/factsheets.html
Columbia University Medical Center's Fact Sheets on Alternative Medicine.

www.dearest.com
This award-winning site is a lively and even magical online women's resource that includes animation and music. The site offers emotional support and features interviews with big names in the menopause field.

Medline: www.ncbi.nlm.nih.gov/Entrez/medline.html
An abundant source of published medical research papers, many with abstracts summarizing the study and the results. It's quick and easy to search and has many cross-references. Enter a search word, then narrow the reference by entering another key word.

menopause-online.com
This site offers information about traditional and complementary treatments. Included is a review of "natural" estrogens and a self-test to evaluate whether postmenopausal estrogen therapy would improve your health profile. There are also many links to other sites and information sources. (If you forget the hyphen, you will come to an anti-Premarin Web site sponsored by PETA [People for the Ethical Treatment of Animals].)

Doctor's Guide to the Internet:
www.pslgroup.com/docguide.htm
Designed to help physicians find resources on the Internet and the World Wide Web. This site provides a great deal of

information from traditional sources on many health issues, including menopause.

altmed.od.nib.gov/nccam
National Institutes of Health's National Center for Complementary Medicine.

Premature Ovarian Failure Support Group:
www.POFSupport.org
This site includes a newsletter, frequently asked questions, and member recommendations.

pslgroup.com/medconf.htm
The Doctor's Guide to Medical Conferences: This site lists conferences all over the world that are searchable using key words to find a specific subject or location.

sph.uth.tmc.edu/utcam/default.htm
University of Texas Center for Alternative Medicine Research.

wellwoman.com
Web site of Molly Siple, one of the authors of this book, featuring pertinent information on women's health as well as healing foods that support long-term health.

Sources for Alternative Medications and Supplements

Biosource Nutrition
P.O. Box 200
Franklin Lakes, NJ 07417
1-800-206-2006
Fax: 1-201-337-0404
www.biosourcenutrition.com
A discount mail-order catalog that offers name-brand nutritional supplements and herbs.

Transitions for Health
621 S.W. Alder, Suite 990
Portland, OR 97205
1-503-226-1010
Makes Pro-Gest cream, topically applied natural progesterone. Independent testing has confirmed that each ounce of
   the cream contains 450 milligrams of progesterone.

Vitamin Shopper
1-800-223-1216
A discount catalog for ordering name-brand herbs and supplements.

Women's International Pharmacy
5708 Monona Drive
Madison, WI 53716
1-800-279-5708
Women's International Pharmacy offers natural progesterone
   pills packed in olive oil. They will send a packet of extensive
   research information on request.

Hormone Replacement Therapies

The following companies produce and/or distribute the three
forms of estrogen, natural progesterone, and DHEA. You will
need to present a doctor's prescription for most of the products. Phone or write for the most recent catalog.

College Pharmacy
833 North Tejon Street
Colorado Springs, CO 80903
1-800-888-9358

Delk Pharmacy
1602 Hatcher Lane
Columbia, TN 38401
1-615-388-3952

Key Pharmacy Compounding Center
23422 Pacific Highway South
Kent, WA 98032
1-800-878-1322
Fax: 1-888-878-1118

Professional and Technical Services
333 Northeast Sandy Boulevard
Portland, OR 97232
1-800-648-8211

Women's International Pharmacy
5708 Monona Drive
Madison, WI 53719-3152
1-800-279-5708

Laboratories Offering Saliva Tests for Hormone Levels

Aeron Biotechnology
1933 Davis Street, Suite 310
San Leandro, CA 94577
1-800-367-3296

Diagnos-Techs, Inc.
6620 South 192nd Place, #J-104
Kent, WA 98032
1-800-87-TESTS or 1-206-251-0596
This laboratory works only with physicians; however, women
can receive information on these tests from Dr. Rebecca
Wunsome. Send for information.

National BioTech Laboratory
3212 N.E. 125th Street
Seattle, WA 98125
1-800-846-6285 or 1-206-363-6606

Urinary Tests for Bone Resorption

Great Smokies Diagnostic Laboratory
18A Regent Park Boulevard
Ashville, NC 28806
1-800-522-4762 or 1-704-253-0621

Meredian Valley Clinical Lab
515 Harrison Street, Suite 9
Kent, WA 98042
1-800-234-6825 or 1-206-859-8700

MetaMatrix Medical Laboratory
5000 Peachtree Ind. Boulevard, Suite 110
Norcross, GA 30071
1-800-221-4640 or 1-404-446-5483

Ostrex International
2203 Airport Way South, Suite 301
Seattle, WA 98134
800-99-OSTEX or 1-206-292-8082

Sources of Organically Grown, Hormone-Free, Nitrite-Free Meat and Poultry

Coleman Natural Beef. Available at supermarkets throughout the United States including Grand Union stores in the
New York City area as well as Purity Supreme in New En-

gland, A&P in New York and New Jersey, Bread & Circus in the Boston area, Big Y Foods in Massachusetts, and Farmer Jack stores in the Detroit, Michigan, area.

Foster Farms poultry is available in most supermarkets throughout the western United States. Has a rigorous pesticide residue elimination program, screening all shipments of grain. Subtherapeutic doses of antibiotics and other drugs are not used.

Fresh Australian Range Lamb is range-fed and raised without the use of hormones and antibiotics. www.amlc.com

Holly Farms poultry is available throughout the eastern and midwestern states. Has a rigorous pesticide residue elimination program. Subtherapeutic doses of antibiotics and other drugs are not used. Found in most supermarkets.

Kohler Farms of Wisconsin supplies hormone-free beef to supermarkets in Wisconsin and the Chicago area including Treasure Island. Look for the PURElean BEEF trademark.

Larsen Beef, produced without antibiotics or hormones, can be found in Kroger stores in Atlanta, Georgia, as well as King Kullen in Long Island, New York, Kash N Karry in the Tampa and Orlando, Florida, areas and Dominicks in the Chicago area.

Laura's Lean Beef, produced without hormones, is available at Kroger stores in Kentucky and southern Indiana.

Maverick Ranch Lite Beef is produced without hormones or antibiotics and is lab tested for pesticide residues. Available at King Supermarkets in Denver, Colorado, Schnucks in Saint Louis, Missouri, Kings Supermarkets in New Jersey, and Clemens in Philadelphia, Pennsylvania.

Organic Cattle Co. beef is certified organic and available at supermarkets in the New York City area.

Quality Steaks produces hormone-free beef that is available at Star Markets in Massachusetts, First National Supermarkets in New England, and ABCO in the Phoenix, Arizona, area.

For Further Reading

Barbach, Lonnie. *The Pause: Positive Approaches to Menopause.* New York: Dutton/Penguin, 1993.

Chopra, Deepak. *Ageless Body, Timeless Mind.* New York: Harmony Books, 1993.

Cobb, Janine O'Leary. *Understanding Menopause.* New York: Penguin, 1994.

De Angelis, Lissa G., and Molly Siple. *Recipes for Change: Gourmet Wholefood Cooking for Health and Vitality at Menopause.* New York: Dutton/Penguin, 1996.

De Angelis, Lissa G., and Molly Siple. *SOS for PMS: Wholefood Solutions for Premenstrual Syndrome.* New York: Plume/Penguin Putnam, 1999.

Erasmus, Udo. *Fats That Heal, Fats That Kill.* Burnaby, BC, Canada: Alive Books, 1993.

Gaby, Alan. *Preventing and Reversing Osteoporosis: Every Woman's Essential Guide.* Rocklin, CA: Prima Publishing, 1994.

Gittleman, Ann Louise. *Supernutrition for Menopause.* New York: Pocket Books, 1993.

Greenwood, Sadja. *Menopause Naturally*, 2nd edition. Volcano, CA: Volcano Press, 1992.

Lark, Susan. *The Menopause Self-Help Book.* Berkeley, CA: Celestial Arts, 1992.

Murray, Michael T. *Menopause: How You Can Benefit from Diet, Vitamins, Minerals, Herbs, Exercise.* Rocklin, CA: Prima Publishing, 1994.

Murray, Michael T., and Joseph Pizzorno. *Encyclopedia of Natural Medicine.* Rocklin, CA: Prima Publishing, 1991.

Northrup, Christiane. *Women's Bodies, Women's Wisdom.* New York: Bantam Books, 1994.

Ojeda, Linda. *Menopause Without Medicine.* Alameda, CA: Hunter House, 1992.

Siple, Molly. *Healing Foods for Dummies.* Foster City, CA: IDG Books Worldwide, 1999.

Weed, Susan. *Menopause Years: The Wise Woman Way.* Woodstock, NY: Ashtree Publishing, 1992.

Weil, Andrew. *Natural Health, Natural Medicine.* Boston: Houghton Mifflin, 1990.

Werback, Melvin. *Healing Through Nutrition.* New York: HarperCollins, 1993.

Index

acidic food and osteoporosis,
   198–199
active relaxation yoga
   posture, 135
adrenal glands
   caffeine and, 86
   role of, 146–147
   stress and, 148–149
aerobic exercise
   benefits of, 138–139
   overview of, 137
alcohol, 199
American Herbal Products
   Association (AHPA), 107
androgens, 31, 171
androstenedione, 12, 147
anger, 27–28
antioxidants, 81
arachidonic acid, 96–97
artificial menopause, 5
Aswini Mudra yoga posture,
   135–136

B-complex vitamins, 50–51
beta-carotene, 49–50
Beyene, Yewoubdar, 19–20
biofeedback, 188
bioflavonoids, 41, 76–77
black cohosh, 42, 103, 110–111
blueberries, 183
body changes, 32
bone loss. *See* osteoporosis
bone mineral density, 195–196
books, recommended, 228–229
boron, 41, 61
brain fog, 30–31
breast cancer, 163, 174–175
breathing, yogic type, 130–131
bromelain, 192
butter, 99

caffeine
   in diet, 85–86
   osteoporosis and, 199–200
   stress and, 151–152

231

calcium
  exercise and, 140
  forms of, 74–75
  osteoporosis and, 199–201
  overview of, 61–62
cancer
  breast type, 163, 174–175
  endometrial type, 167
  uterine type, 169
carotenoids, 49–50
chamomile, 42, 115, 152
charting symptoms, 37–38,
  39, 40
chasteberry, 116
Chinese medicine, 103–104,
  136
cholesterol, 190–191, 193
chromium, 62–63
Climara, 161
cobalamin (B_{12}), 55–56
colas, 85–86
contraindications for pill form
  of estrogen, 159–160
copper, 63–64
cramps, 96–97, 124
cranberries, 183–184
cultural issues, 14, 17–18, 153
cystitis, 183

dandelion, 185
decoction, 103–104
depression, 6, 28, 124
diary. *See* journal
diet
  cholesterol, 190–191
  colas, 85–86

fats and oils, 98–99
fiber, 85
fish and shellfish, 97
heart disease and, 190
improving, 86, 99–100
incontinence and, 187
legumes, 92
meat and poultry, 96–97
organic food, 89–90
osteoporosis and, 198–200
overview of, 41, 83–84
plant food, 88–89
resources for, 226–228
stress management and,
  150–152
sugar, 84–85, 151
symptoms and, 20
traditional vs. modern, 87
urinary tract infection and,
  183–184
vegetables and fruit, 92–95
whole foods, 86–87
whole grains, 90–91, 191
dioxin, 90
disease and aging
  heart disease, 189–193
  incontinence, 185–188
  osteoporosis, 193–203
  overview of, 179–180
  thyroid problems, 180–182
  urinary tract infection,
    182–185
doctor
  alternative health
    professionals, 217–218
  herbs and, 105, 106–107

dong quai, 42, 108–109
drugs
  herbs compared to, 101–103
  interactions with, 175
  See also medication
dual-energy x-ray
    absorptiometer (DEXA),
    195

echinacea, 185
emotions
  anger, 27–28
  anxiety, irritability, 123
  depression, 6, 28, 124
  exercise for, 142
  hot flashes and, 24
  mood swings, 26–27, 123
  stress and, 145–146
endometrial cancer, 167
Environmental Working
    Group, 94
essential fatty acids, 80–81,
    97
Ester-C ascorbate, 73
Estrace, 156
Estraderm, 161
estradiol, 78, 159–160
Estratab, 160
estriol, 12, 111, 163
estrogen
  emotions and, 26
  hot flashes and, 23–24
  menopause and, 11–12
  menstrual cycle and, 7
  osteoporosis and, 172
  purpose of, 9–10

stress hormones and, 147
verbal memory and, 30
estrogen replacement therapy
  benefits of, 157
  breast cancer and, 174–175
  dosage, 160, 161, 162–163
  forms of, 159–164
  heart disease and, 172–174,
    189–190
  history of, 156
  osteoporosis and, 196–197
  progesterone, combining
    with, 169–170
  side effects, 164–165
  types of, 158
estrone, 12, 147, 160
estropipate, 162
exercise
  aerobic type, 137–140
  benefits of, 127–128
  forms of, 128
  heart disease and, 191–192
  incorporating into daily
    routine, 141
  osteoporosis and, 139–140,
    201–202
  overview of, 42
  pace of, 140–141
  qigong, 136
  starting, 129
  stress management and,
    154
  tai chi, 136–137
  urinary tract infection and,
    185
  yoga, 129–136

false unicorn root, 116–117
fatigue, 25–26, 123, 142
fats, 98–99, 190
female reproductive organs, 7
fiber, 85
fish and shellfish, 97
flaxseed, 79–80
flaxseed oil, 99
flour, refined, 151
fluid retention, 125
folic acid, 56–57
follicle-stimulating hormone
    (FSH)
  measuring level of, 175–176
  menstrual cycle and, 7
  purpose of, 9–10
forward bending yoga
    postures, 133–134
Fosamax, 202–203
free radicals, 81
fruits, 92–93, 94–95

garden sage, 120–121
gingko biloba, 117–118
ginseng
  oriental or panax, 111–112
  Siberian, 112–113
glands influencing
    menopause, 8
glucose, 84–85
goldenseal, 185

hawthorne berries, 192
health organizations, 213–217
health research, 9
heart disease

  cholesterol and, 190–191,
    193
  exercise and, 191–192
  fat intake and, 190
  healing foods, 191
  herbs for, 192
  hormone replacement
    therapy and, 172–174
  hypertension, 191
  overview of, 189–190
  testing for, 192–193
heart palpitations, 22
heavy menstrual bleeding,
    3, 125
herbs
  black cohosh, 42, 103,
    110–111
  chamomile, 42, 115, 152
  chasteberry, 116
  dong quai, 42, 108–109
  drugs compared to, 101–103
  expiration date, 106
  false unicorn root, 116–117
  forms of, 103–104
  garden sage, 120–121
  gingko biloba, 117–118
  ginseng, 111–113
  heart disease and, 192
  incontinence and, 187
  licorice, 118–119
  manufacturer, calling, 107
  motherwort, 119–120, 185
  osteoporosis and, 202
  overview of, 42, 101–102,
    108
  potency of, 105–106

red clover, 77, 113–115
sarsaparilla, 121–122
side effects, 105
by signs of menopause,
    122–125
sources of, 106
urinary tract infection and,
    184–185
using safely, 104–105, 107
valerian, 122
homeopathy and physical well-
    being, 2
hormone replacement therapy
    benefits of, 157–158
    breast cancer and, 174–175
    combining estrogen with
        progesterone, 169–170
    disease prevention and,
        171–174, 189–190
    drug interactions, 175
    estrogen supplement,
        158–165
    goal of, 176–177
    history of, 156
    osteoporosis and, 196–197
    overview of, 43–44,
        155–156
    progesterone supplement,
        165–168
    resources for, 224–225
    side effects, 164–165,
        168–169
    testosterone, 170–171
hormones
    adrenal glands and, 146–147
    black cohosh and, 110–111

measuring levels of, 175–176,
    225–226
meat and, 97
menopause and, 15
menstrual cycle and, 7
negative feedback system, 9
perimenopause and, 10–11
sex type, 10
specialty pharmacies as
    source of, 163–164
thyroid problems and,
    181–182
hot flashes
    breathing and, 130–131
    chemistry of, 23–24
    description of, 21–22
    emotional reaction to, 24
    exercise for, 142
    herbs for, 122–123
    night sweats and, 24–25
    stress and, 145–146
    timing of, 22–23
HRT. See hormone
    replacement therapy
hypertension, 191
hypothalamus, 23

incontinence. See urinary
    incontinence
infusion, 103
insecticides, 89–90
inverted yoga postures,
    132–133
iodine, 64, 181
iron, 64–65
isoflavones, 114

Japanese experience, 17–18, 78–79

journal
  associating symptoms and activities in, 37
  charting symptoms in, 37–38, 39, 40
  overview of, 36–37, 38

Kegel exercises, 186–187

lean cuts of meat, 96
legumes, 92
libido, 124, 170
licorice, 118–119
lifestyle and osteoporosis, 197–198
low-fat diet, 190
low-impact aerobic exercise, 138–139
luteinizing hormone (LH)
  menstrual cycle and, 7
  purpose of, 9–10

magnesium, 65–66, 199, 201
manganese, 66–67
meat and poultry, 96–97, 226–228
medication
  osteoporosis, 202–203
  thyroid problems, 182
  See also drugs
meditation, 152–153
medroxyprogesterone acetate, 166
melatonin, 25

memory loss
  exercise for, 142
  herbs for, 124
  overview of, 29–30
menopause
  approach to, 15–16
  conversation about, 1
  cultural issues, 14, 17–18, 153
  social issues in, 12–14
  statistics on, 6
  types of, 5–6
  varying course of, 1–2, 4
menorrhagia, 158
menstrual bleeding, 3, 125
menstrual cycle, 6–8, 125
micronized progesterone, 167
midlife stress, 149–150
minerals
  boron, 61
  calcium, 61–62, 74–75, 140, 199–201
  chromium, 62–63
  copper, 63–64
  fish and shellfish, 97
  iodine, 64, 181
  iron, 64–65
  magnesium, 65–66, 199, 201
  manganese, 66–67
  overview of, 60
  phosphorus, 67–68
  potassium, 68, 191
  recommendations for, 71–72
  selenium, 68–69, 97
  zinc, 69–70

mood swings, 26–27, 123, 142
motherwort, 119–120, 185

natural estrogen, 158, 162,
    163–164
natural hormones, 163–164
natural menopause, 5
natural progesterone, 166–168
niacin (B$_3$), 53–54
night sweats, 24, 122–123
19-nortestosterone compound,
    166
norepinephrine, 23
nutrients
  bioflavonoids, 41, 76–77
  essential fatty acids, 80–81
  food sources vs. supplements,
    48
  form of key types of,
    73–75
  osteoporosis and, 199–200
  overview of, 38, 41, 47
  phytoestrogens, 41, 77–80
  stress management and,
    150–152
  symptoms and, 82
  urinary tract infection and,
    184
  See also minerals; vitamins

Ogen, 156, 160
oils, 98–99
omega-3 fatty acid, 97
organic food
  benefits of, 89–90
  resources for, 226–228

organs influencing menopause,
    8
oriental ginseng, 111–112
osteoporosis
  acidic food and, 198–199
  bone density and, 194–196
  colas and, 86
  exercise and, 142, 201–202
  herbs and, 202
  hormone replacement ther-
    apy and, 171–172, 196–197
  lifestyle and, 197–198
  medication for, 202–203
  overview of, 193–194
  prevention of, 134–135, 136,
    139–140
  stress and, 202
  supplements for, 200–201
  urinary tests for bone
    resorption, 226

panax ginseng, 111–112
pantothenic acid (B$_5$), 54
patch form of estrogen, 161
perimenopause, 3, 10–11
pesticides, 89–90, 94–95
phosphorus, 67–68
physician
  alternative health
    professionals, 217–218
  herbs and, 105, 106–107
phytoestrogens
  effects of, 78–79
  food sources of, 79–80
  importance of, 78
  overview of, 41, 77

phytohormones, 167

piezoelectric effect, 139

pill form of estrogen, 159–160

plant food, 88–89

postures for yoga
  active relaxing, 135
  forward bends, 133–134
  inversions, 132–133
  overview of, 131–132
  subtle movements, 135–136
  twists, 134
  weight-bearing, 134–135

potassium, 68, 191

prana, 133

Premarin, 156, 159, 160, 162,
  163–164

premature menopause, 5–6

produce, shopping for, 92–93

Progest, 168

progesterone
  dosage, 166, 167–168
  emotions and, 26
  estrogen, combining with,
    169–170
  forms of, 166–168
  menstrual cycle and, 7
  osteoporosis and, 172, 197
  purpose of, 9–10
  side effects, 168–169
  as supplement, 157–158
  types of, 165–166

progestin, 165–166

protein, 96–97

pyridoxine (B_6), 55

qigong, 128, 136

red clover, 77, 113–115

refined grain, 91, 151

REM (rapid eye movement)
  sleep, 150

research, 9

resources
  alternative health
    professionals, 217–218
  alternative medications and
    supplements, 223–224
  books, 228–229
  health organizations,
    213–217
  hormone replacement
    therapy, 224–225
  newsletters and publications,
    218–221
  phone numbers, 218
  saliva tests for hormone
    levels, 225–226
  specialty pharmacies,
    163–164
  urinary tests for bone
    resorption, 226
  Web pages, 222–223

riboflavin (B_2), 52–53

sage, garden type, 120–121

saponins, 102

sarsaparilla, 121–122

selenium, 68–69, 97

self-acceptance, 15

Selye, Hans, 148

sex hormones
  overview of, 10
  stress hormones and, 147

sexuality
  libido, 124, 170
  menopause and, 6, 31–32
Siberian ginseng, 112–113
side effects
  estrogen replacement
    therapy, 164–165
  progesterone, 168–169
signs
  anger, 27–28
  brain fog, 30–31
  change in profile, 29
  depression, 6, 28, 124
  fatigue, 25–26, 123, 142
  hot flashes, 21–25, 122–123,
    142, 145–146
  memory loss, 29–30, 124, 142
  mood swings, 26–27, 123, 142
  overview of, 21
  sexuality, 31, 124
  symptoms compared
    to, 20
  weight gain, 28–29
Six-Step Healthy Menopause
  Program
  benefits of, 35–36
  compliance with, 44–45
  diet, 41
  exercise, 42
  herbs, 42
  hormone replacement
    therapy, 43–44
  journal and, 36–38
  nutrients, 38, 41
  overview of, 3
  stress management, 42–43

sleep problems, night sweats
  and, 24–25, 149–150
social issues, 12–14
sodium, 191
soybeans, 114
specialty pharmacies, 163–164
standardized preparation,
  105–106
steroidal saponin, 102
steroid hormones, 10
stress
  adrenal glands and, 146–147,
    148–149
  benefits of, 148
  midlife period and, 149–150
  osteoporosis and, 202
  overview of, 145–146
  stages of, 148–149
  See also stress management
stress management
  chamomile and, 152
  exercise and, 154
  foods to avoid, 151–152
  meditation, 152–153
  overview of, 42–43, 150–151
  positive imagery, 153–154
  techniques for, 152
sugar, 84–85, 151
supplements
  food sources compared to, 48
  nutrient ratios, 70–71
  osteoporosis and, 200–201
  overview of, 70
  recommendations for, 71–72
  resources for, 223–224
surgical menopause, 5

Symptom Frequency Chart, 39
symptoms
  charting, 37–38, 39, 40
  cultural factors in, 17–18
  disease compared to, 33–34
  signs compared to, 20
  variability in, 18–20
Symptom Trigger Chart, 40
synthetic estrogen, 158
synthetic progesterone, 165–166

tai chi, 128, 136–137
tea, herbal type, 103
testosterone, 170–171
thiamin (B_1), 51–52
thyroid gland
  adrenal glands and, 146
  medication for, 182
  problems with, 180
  testing, 180–181
  therapies for, 181–182
tincture, 104
transdermal estrogen, 161
trans-fatty acid, 99
Tri-Est, 163
triglyceride level, 193
twisting yoga postures, 134

unrefined oil, 98–99
urinary incontinence
  dealing with, 187
  estrogen and, 157
  foods and, 187
  herbs and, 187
  Kegel exercises, 186–187
  overview of, 185–186
  treating, 188
urinary tract infection
  diet and healing foods, 183–184
  exercise and, 185
  herbs for, 184–185
  medication for, 185
  nutrients for, 184
  overview of, 182–183
U.S. Pharmacopeia, 106
uterine cancer, 169
uva ursi, 185

vagina, changes in, 32, 124, 142
vaginal cream form of estrogen, 161–163
vaginitis, 32–33
valerian, 122
varicose veins, 76
vegetables, 92–93, 94–95
vegetarian diet, 88
vitamins
  A, 49–50
  B-complex, 50–51
  beta-carotene, 49–50
  C, 57–58, 73
  cobalamin (B_{12}), 55–56
  D, 58
  E, 59, 73–74
  folic acid, 56–57
  meat and poultry, 96
  niacin (B_3), 53–54
  overview of, 48–49

pantothenic acid (B$_5$), 54
pyridoxine (B$_6$), 55
recommendations for, 71–72
riboflavin (B$_2$), 52–53
thiamin (B$_1$), 51–52
volatile oil, 102

walking, 129
Web pages, 222–223
weight-bearing exercise
  benefits of, 139–140
  osteoporosis and, 201–202
  overview of, 137
  yoga postures, 134–135
weight gain, 28–29
whole food, 86–87
whole grains, 90–91, 191

yoga
  active relaxing postures,
    135
  benefits of, 128
  breathing and, 130–131
  forward bending postures,
    133–134
  inversion postures, 132–133
  overview of, 129–130
  postures, 131–132
  subtle movements, 135–136
  twisting postures, 134
  weight-bearing postures,
    134–135

zinc, 69–70